I0827707

Unburied

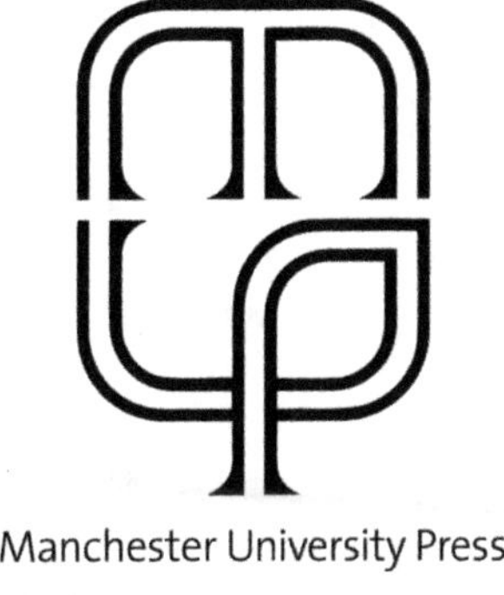

Manchester University Press

Unburied

The true story of Hannah Beswick, the Manchester Mummy

Hannah Priest

Manchester University Press

Published by Manchester University Press
Oxford Road, Manchester, M13 9PL

www.manchesteruniversitypress.co.uk

British Library Cataloguing-in-Publication Data
A catalogue record for this book is available from the British Library

ISBN 978 1 5261 7592 2 hardback

First published 2025

Typeset by Newgen Publishing UK

For Hannah
Rest in Peace

Contents

Acknowledgements

It's always tempting for a writer to claim credit for unburying their sources, particularly for a story that hasn't been told before. In truth, the sources I used to piece together Hannah Beswick's story weren't buried, but rather preserved and catalogued by archivists and librarians. I would particularly like to thank staff at the John Rylands Research Institute and Library, University of Manchester Library, Manchester Libraries Archives+ and Oldham Libraries for their assistance and advice as I put Hannah's story together. I would also like to thank staff at Chetham's Library for persevering with finding some source material, even when it appeared that a certain diary was cursed. I hope everything's okay.

Thank you to Lancashire Archives and Borthwick Institute for Archives at the University of York for scanning so many wills and probate documents for me, and to the many, many people who have contributed work and services to building the British Newspaper Archive, without which this book would have been much harder to write, and I probably still wouldn't know where to hire a hearse in eighteenth-century Manchester.

I would also like to thank Jolene Zigarovich and Kate Ash-Irisarri for their assistance with locating specific academic sources. The help was very gratefully received.

Prologue

> In 1835, Manchester's Natural History Society opened its museum on Peter Street. On display in the museum were three mummies. One was an Ancient Egyptian mummy. One was a Peruvian mummy. And one was an old woman from Hollinwood, who'd been mummified by her family doctor and put on display to the public. And you thought your GP was bad …

You may already know about the story of Hannah Beswick, the so-called 'Manchester Mummy', or perhaps this is the first time you've heard about it. A wealthy woman from Manchester, Hannah was mummified by her doctor and placed in a museum collection. In the nineteenth century, her body was displayed in the museum of Manchester's Natural History Society, the precursor institution to the Manchester Museum, where it sat alongside Egyptian and Peruvian mummies. The reasons behind her curious fate are a source of speculation, with the main theories being that either she was terrified of being buried alive, or the doctor had more sinister reasons for preventing the woman's burial.

I first came across the story of Hannah Beswick in 2015. Under the name Hannah Kate, I present a weekly literature show on my local community radio station, North Manchester FM. In October 2015, when the show was relatively new, I decided to do a Halloween Special, which would feature a number of local (i.e. North Manchester) ghost stories. My search for quirky tales led me to the story of Hannah Beswick, which I duly recounted on air. I talked about the mummification, the woman's fear of being buried alive, and some of the suggestions that her doctor may have been behaving badly. I also explained that Hannah Beswick was, eventually, buried in an unmarked grave in Harpurhey Cemetery, a municipal graveyard just a couple of minutes' walk away from the North Manchester FM studios. Following the burial, a number of hauntings were reported around the site of Hannah Beswick's old house in Hollinwood, near Oldham, including sightings of a grey lady (sometimes headless) at the Ferranti factory that was built on the land. Some versions of the story state that Hannah Beswick hid gold in her house before her death, and that the ghostly apparitions are the woman searching for, or protecting, her lost treasure.

This was a performance, of course, so I couldn't help but add my own flourish to the story. I ended my version of the tale by saying that if you go to the far corner of Harpurhey Cemetery, and you find just the right spot, where an unmarked grave sits underneath a tree, and you're very, very quiet, you might just make out the sound of fingernails scraping against wood, and a voice saying, 'I'm not dead yet.'

I claimed this last bit as local legend but, in fact, it was my own invention, a little bit of extra Halloween spookiness to finish up my performance. I performed the story again at a number of events in subsequent months, and in 2018 I was asked to contribute a Hannah Beswick-inspired piece to an anthology called *The Spooky Isles Book of Horror*. My story was called 'Dust to Dust', and it featured a group of wannabe ghosthunters in Hollinwood falling victim to the vengeful spirit of Hannah Beswick, who ends the tale by stating (via the young woman she has possessed), 'I'm not dead yet.' The story was followed by a short essay about the historical background that inspired the creative piece.

At the same time, under the name Hannah Priest, I had started giving local history talks around Manchester, and so I developed a talk on Hannah Beswick to include in my portfolio. The connections to familiar locations in North Manchester and Oldham, coupled with the inherent creepy weirdness of the story, made it one of my most popular talks.

Although the local history talks I give are a little more serious and contain more references than my creative output, they are still performances of a kind. My Hannah Beswick talk may have debunked some elements of the story (including the claim that the woman left instructions in her will that her body should be kept above ground), but it still played on the spookiness of the story, not least in my choice of PowerPoint font, chosen to resemble a horror film poster. I included a description of the likely preservation techniques used by the doctor, which was always guaranteed to get a shudder from the audience. And I talked about the ghost sightings around Hollinwood, which would usually get a nod of recognition from audience members who knew the places mentioned or a giggle as I recounted some of the wilder activities of the alleged ghost. The talk always began with the same opening lines, the ones I've included at the beginning of this prologue, which usually raised at least a small laugh from the audience. It's such a bizarre story, with elements ranging from the macabre museum to the Gothic fear of premature burial and the sinister medical man with a hidden agenda, that it always provoked interest.

I was booked to give the talk at the Manchester branch of the National Trust in April 2020. This event was, of course, postponed due to the national COVID-19 lockdown.

In April 2022, I stood in front of the audience to give my rescheduled talk, horror-styled PowerPoint projected onto a screen behind me. I clicked onto my first slide, a sketch of the Peter Street museum, and I gave my opening lines, 'In 1835, Manchester's Natural History Society opened its museum on Peter Street …' And I got the usual laugh when I said, 'And one was an old woman from Hollinwood …'

But then something happened.

I can't explain why it happened, but I have to assume it was a reaction to everything that had gone on over the previous two years of COVID-19 and lockdown. Something in me had shifted, and I just couldn't look at the story I was presenting in the same way.

I gave the talk in its usual format (the group had booked me to do that, after all), but all I could think as I spoke was that this woman I was describing, Hannah Beswick, was a human being, a real person who had lived and died not far from where I live now. She may be known now only for the manner of her post-mortem preservation and spectral appearances, but she was once a living, breathing person.

I came out of the talk with the absolute conviction that it was time I got to know Hannah Beswick better. I knew it wouldn't be easy, as every account of the Manchester Mummy I'd read at that point either omitted details of the woman's life or dismissed it as 'unremarkable'. But it was still a life, and I wanted to know more about it.

In many ways, I find myself in the same position as I was in at Halloween 2015. I still want to tell the story of Hannah Beswick. It's just that now I want to tell you the true story.

Part I

Afterlife

1
The cabinet of insects

There are a number of places where we could start this story, but let's begin here: with a cabinet of insects.

The cabinet in question was actually three large mahogany showcases filled with hundreds of preserved insects that had been collected by a man named John Leigh Philips, a mill owner and industrialist in eighteenth-century Manchester whose father had founded the cotton-spinning company Philips and Lee. The insects, along with other natural history specimens, had been displayed in Philips's house for any interested visitors. This may seem like a strange place to begin to explain the Manchester Mummy – a tale that has come to be both ghost story and urban legend – but Philips's collection plays a significant role in understanding what happened to the mummy, and so this is where we start.

A 'cabinet', strictly speaking, was a room (or rooms) in a private premises used to house a collection of noteworthy or interesting objects. But as the practice of collecting developed, it would come to mean both the furniture within the display room and the collection itself. You may have heard the term 'cabinet of curiosities', but there was a difference between a 'cabinet' collection – which would include objects of scientific or practical significance, such as specimens from the plant and animal kingdoms, sketches and illustrations, mineral and rock samples, etc. – and a 'curiosities' collection – which might include items chosen for their exoticism, strangeness or other aesthetic qualities.

One of the most significant collectors in eighteenth-century Britain was the physician Hans Sloane. His collection of plant and animal specimens, cultural and ethnological artifacts, minerals, shells and other notable items, including hundreds of books and additional cabinets purchased from other collectors, was bequeathed to the nation on his death in 1753 and became the basis for the British Museum. Closer to home, for the purposes of our story, was the cabinet of Ashton Lever. Lever was born at Alkrington Hall near Middleton (around four miles from what is now the centre of Manchester) in 1729, the son of Sir James Darcy Lever, who served as High Sheriff of Lancashire. He began his interest in natural history by collecting live birds, which he housed in an expansive aviary at his family home on his return from Oxford. When he was in his early thirties, he sold his birds and began acquiring shells and fossils, and by 1766 he'd put together a vast collection of natural history specimens that filled over 1,000 display cases. Lever first opened up his cabinet for public viewing at his house on Lever's Row (now Piccadilly) in Manchester, and later at Alkrington Hall, where local legend tells us he kept a pet wolf as one of his 'curiosities'. When he moved to London in 1774, his cabinet was exhibited there, and he continued to purchase objects for it until he faced bankruptcy.

The cabinet of John Leigh Philips had neither the cultural magnitude of Hans Sloane's cabinet, nor the flamboyant panache of Ashton Lever's. It was, on the whole, a collection of assiduously catalogued insects. However, it left a legacy in Manchester that has been experienced and enjoyed by countless thousands of residents and visitors.

When John Leigh Philips died in 1814, his collection – which had previously been a personal endeavour, shared with scholars and other interested parties on request – was put up for sale. The advertisement that ran in the *Manchester Meteor* promised a 'valuable, extensive and well-chosen library' that covered a wide range of subjects from divinity to typography, natural history, rural sports and experimental philosophy, plus some rare English and French novels. It also included 'the valuable and nearly complete CABINET of INSECTS, formed by the late J. L. Philips, esq. with unremitting attention in a period of near thirty years, scientifically arranged, and in the most perfect state of preservation. And many other valuable Specimens of Natural History'.[1] Although the library appears to have been broken up and sold piecemeal via a catalogue that cost two shillings itself to purchase, the cabinet of insects (the mahogany cases of entomological specimens) was bought by Thomas Henry Robinson. Robinson was a member of Manchester's Literary and Philosophical Society, as Philips had been, and his newly acquired cabinet was likely housed in his private residence, as it had been in Philips's. Records of the sale have not survived, but the entire collection appears to have been sold for over £5,000.[2]

The Manchester Lit and Phil was founded in 1781 and is the second oldest surviving scientific society in England, after the Royal Society. Prior to the formation of the Manchester Mechanics' Institute in 1824 and Owens College in 1851, the Lit and Phil was the pre-eminent scholarly organization in the city, with membership drawn from the city's 'new and increasingly wealthy elite' of manufacturers, inventors, chemists, lawyers and – increasingly – physicians.[3] Thomas Henry Robinson, a man who, like many members of the society, was both a cotton merchant and a Unitarian, served as Secretary from 1817 to 1822.[4]

In 1821, Robinson offered Philips's cabinet of insects for sale to the Lit and Phil, to augment the already large library the organization had built up and, presumably, the city's subscription newsroom and library, the Portico Library, which opened its doors to subscribers in 1806 and shared membership with the Lit and Phil.

The society declined to buy the cabinet of insects.

This decision isn't a particularly surprising one. In the early nineteenth century, 'cabinets' still retained their status as private collections, to be housed in residential properties by individuals and opened only to invited guests (with the exception of the collections of more idiosyncratic individuals, such as Ashton Lever, which might be opened to the public). They were distinct from libraries and, for some, less worthy objects of scholarly attention. Cabinets of curiosities – or wonder-rooms, *Wunderkammern* – featured in sideshows and fairs as much as in intellectual societies, and were the precursor to, for instance, Barnum's American Museum, which opened in 1841. While

Philips's mahogany cases of perfectly preserved insects are rarely compared to the attractions created by P. T. Barnum, they do grow out of the same tradition of individual curation and display, rather than the collective and collaborative work of a group of scholars.

There may also have been practical reasons for the Lit and Phil's decision to turn down Robinson's offer. If the society had taken on the cabinet, then a home would have been needed for it, and members would have had the responsibility not only for housing the collection, but also for allowing access for approved visitors. Interestingly, other urban literary and philosophical societies would take a different approach to Manchester. Both the Sheffield and Hull societies were formed in 1822, and from the start these organizations included collections of natural history specimens within their holdings.[5]

The official position of the Manchester society was that it would not enter into the business of specimen collection and curation, but it is clear that not all members agreed with this approach. At a meeting of the Lit and Phil in 1821 – possibly the same meeting at which Robinson suggested transferring his cabinet to society ownership, though some have suggested this may have been a more clandestine breakaway meeting of 'contumacious' members – a group of men proposed the formation of a new society that would be called the Manchester Society for the Promotion of Natural History. This new society would share membership with the Lit and Phil, but its focus would be different.

The new Manchester Society for the Promotion of Natural History quickly raised funds and purchased Robinson's (formerly Philips's) cabinet of insects. They housed the collection in premises on St Ann's Place in Manchester, rented from one of the members.[6] This was the new society's first 'museum', a location in which objects were displayed for the purposes of preservation and contemplation, differing from the previous 'cabinet' in that it was collectively, rather than individually, owned and managed. It was accessible only by members of the society, who contributed financially and encouraged further donations to the collection, which quickly expanded to include ornithological specimens (some of which may have originated in Philips's collection), minerals and crystals, and antiquities. Members of the society paid a £10 per year subscription, a sum which ensured the exclusivity of the establishment as well as its survival.

The increasing size of the society's collection required new premises, and the museum (still a members-only institution) relocated to a two-storey premises in King Street in 1824, where the collection soon acquired a new type of artefact: human remains.

* * *

In 1825, when the Natural History Society were congratulating themselves on having over eight hundred pounds in the bank, as well as annual receipts of over three hundred guineas, the 'beautiful cabinet of insects' was being regularly augmented by donations from both society members and wealthy businessmen of the town.[7] Among the donations from 'gentlemen having commercial establishments abroad' were items from Robert and William Garnett, the sons of John Garnett, a former trader of enslaved people who settled in Manchester to work as a cotton merchant.[8] The Garnett brothers, also cotton merchants, donated an Ancient Egyptian mummy and two associated coffins to the society's collection, along with a crocodile and a 'species of lizard' (both stuffed, one assumes). While it's not clear if these were the first human remains to be deposited with the society, they were certainly the most significant. The mummy, then known as Asroni, was unwrapped in the King Street museum in April 1825.

> The mummy was opened in the presence of the council, and several members of the Society, and the following were some of the appearances noticed:
>
> On taking off the top of the inner case, the body was found covered with a cloth of coarse texture, and of a light brown colour, the removal of which exposed to view a variety of bandages of the same material, passing round the body in different directions, so as to envelope it in an immense number of folds. The inner bandages were very much impregnated with bituminous or resinous matter, of a dark colour, which rendered the cloth so brittle, that the inner folds were obliged to be broken off in pieces.
>
> When the body was exposed, it presented a dark brown appearance, the soft parts being quite shrivelled and dried upon the bones. It was 4 feet 11¾ inches in length, was extremely light, and several of the teeth,

> the finger and toe nails, were quite perfect. The scull, and head altogether, were remarkable for their excellent proportions. On the body were found, in several places, the *larvae* of insects, and a few specimens of a small green coleopterous insect. Under the upper part of the body, on the bottom of the inner case or coffin, a quantity of blue porcelain beads was found, strung on threads in rows, and to them were appended two small square plates, one of them composed of blue porcelaine, the other of a soft kind of stone, both bearing inscriptions.
>
> The bandages were not applied with any great degree of nicety; the cloth was easily torn, and on it no figures or hieroglyphicks were delineated, except at the end of a portion lying on the breast.[9]

The first recorded medical dissection of an Egyptian mummy in Europe was in 1763, and from this there followed a trend for dissecting, unwrapping and displaying displaced bodies for the edification and scientific scrutiny (but also often for the entertainment) of audiences.[10] Asroni was one such displaced body, taken from 'Upper Egypt' by an unknown party, acquired by the Garnetts, stripped of its funeral wrappings under the inspection of the Natural History Society and then displayed in the holdings of the King Street museum. Asroni – now known as Asru – remains in the collection of the Manchester Museum, the successor institution (in some respects) to the Natural History Society's museum, and continues to form a cornerstone of both the antiquities collection at the museum and the ongoing discourse around museology, bioethics and the 'ownership' of human remains.[11]

However, I am getting ahead of myself. To return to King Street, it is clear that the Natural History Society's museum was not simply expanding in the 1820s, but also gaining a reputation as an intellectual institution. While there is only scant information remaining about the society's King Street premises, the testimony of one visitor, George Head, does survive. Head visited the museum in 1834 – the final year it was housed at King Street – and described it as 'one of the best establishments of that nature in England'.[12]

The 'establishments of that nature' to which Head refers are the society museums that were formed in the late eighteenth and early nineteenth centuries by groups of wealthy professional men, usually in urban centres, for the promotion of scholarly pursuits. Museum historian Samuel Alberti identifies two waves in the history of such societies. In the late eighteenth century, there was a wave of Literary and Philosophical Societies (such as Manchester's, which is the oldest surviving example, being formed in 1781 and still in existence at the time of writing), subscriber associations who, in some cases, held small collections of natural history specimens and other artefacts, but who were more focused on 'libraries and lecture series'. And then in the 1820s, a 'second generation' emerged, as a number of regional societies formed with a clearer remit around the foundation of museums, or the holding of collections in 'shared proprietary ownership' (different from the cabinets of individual collectors such as Hans Sloane, Ashton Lever and, indeed, John Leigh Philips). That George Head had seen enough 'establishments of that nature' to attempt a meaningful comparison is evidence of the 'staggering' and 'rapid' growth of such societies in the newly industrialized urban centres of England.[13]

Although Head's work is generally about a tour in 1835, he explains that he actually visited the museum the previous year. Since his visit, he says, the society has moved to new premises, and we'll be turning our attention to those premises shortly. However, we need to stay at King Street for a little longer, as Head's account of his visit reveals something that is of vital significance to our story.

At some point between 1825 and 1834, further human remains had been donated to the Manchester Natural History Society. And when Head visited their museum, Asroni was no longer the only mummy in town.

> Two contrasted specimens of the ancient and modern art of embalming were placed in singular juxta-position with each other; the one the mummy of a female, supposed to have been young, from Thebes, and prepared nobody knows by whom; the other the corpse of an old maiden lady of Manchester, preserved by a late Dr White.[14]

The mummy from Thebes is Asroni, who was then 'supposed to have been young'. Nearly two centuries of research on this body has seen it renamed to Asru (the result of a reinterpretation of inscriptions on the associated coffins) and reassessed as being 50–60 years old at the time of death. Asru is the most studied body in the collection at the Manchester Museum, which means that curators now know her name, occupation (temple chantress), her mother's name (Ta-du-Amen), the effects of her osteoarthritis, the type of cyst in her lung, the type of tapeworm in her body and the type of aromatic oils with which her head was anointed when she was mummified. Asru's head has been reconstructed; her tissue has been stored on the International Egyptian Mummy Tissue Bank (set up at the Manchester Museum in 1997); and her fingerprints have been taken by Greater Manchester Police.

The mummy of the woman from Manchester became a ghost story and urban legend and is, as you might have guessed, the subject of this book.

* * *

When he viewed the bodies in 1834, Head seems to have been most taken with the contrast between the two, as well as the comparison offered between 'the ancient and modern art of embalming':

> The Egyptian damsel lay entirely divested of her cerements; the colours of her portrait within the centre wooden case perfectly vivid, and bundles of blue bugles and coarse linen cloth in good preservation.
>
> The old maid stood upright in a glass case, not in fashionable costume, but enveloped from head to foot, in a dress of blue striped ticking, leaving no part of her person but her face visible, and fitting her so tightly, that it is probable the doctor first paid her over from top to toe with hot glue, and then drew on her garment.[15]

Head's description of this exhibit begins by using the words 'mummy' and 'corpse' to describe the two artefacts, possibly showing an awareness of the specific meaning of the word 'mummy'. The word comes from *mumiya* or *mummia*, terms used in Persian and Arabic to refer to a form of medicinal bitumen (from *mum*, meaning wax), and it came to be associated with preserved Egyptian bodies due to an erroneous idea that the bodies had been preserved with bitumen. The term 'mummy', certainly for some, referred to the embalming products used to preserve the body, rather than a body itself.[16] However, for others, the term came to mean a particular compound formed by the combining of embalming products with the dead body itself, leading to the idea of 'mummification', or the transmutation of the human corpse into another substance through the ritualized application of certain chemicals.[17]

Head's initial introduction of the two bodies on display in the King Street museum makes this distinction: one is a 'mummy', because it has been preserved with Ancient Egyptian mummification practices and associated chemicals, the other is simply a 'preserved corpse'. As we'll see in subsequent chapters, this distinction has not always been made in accounts of viewing human remains in various museums, and the term 'mummy' would come to be applied to a variety of specimens, including embalmed (in a more modern sense), desiccated and taxidermized corpses, sometimes for marketing purposes and sometimes for more poetic reasons.

Although Head's account is initially keen to draw a distinction between the material reality of the two exhibits on display, this indeed quickly gives way to a more poetic assessment. The writer can't help but draw a comparison between the bodies and, furthermore, he appears to have been unable to avoid humanizing them and seeing them specifically as *women*. He goes on to say:

> [T]hey afforded jointly, at least, a curious instance, with regard to the question of age, as to which ladies are said to be particular, that notwithstanding the services of the toilet were in both cases protracted beyond the grave, a difference even of three thousand years certainly was not perceptible.[18]

This assessment of the two embalmed bodies is really rather remarkable. Head not only imagines them as 'ladies', but also hints that they may be happy with that fact that, due to the 'services of the toilet' (a surprisingly genteel euphemism for post-mortem preservation), their respective ages have been obscured.

In considering the stories of Egyptian mummies in museums, Angela Stienne gives numerous examples of how the 'viewing of real people, dead or alive' carried 'an insidious political message'. It encouraged the viewer to believe that 'some people were not just different – they were inferior'. Egyptian mummies, she argues, became key figures in a 'sordid display of racism and othering'.[19]

There are any number of examples of the 'othering' of Egyptian remains to which Stienne refers. However, I am struck by the fact that the earliest description we have of Asru (then Asroni) in the museum is one of domestication rather than exoticization. And it's impossible not to wonder if this is the result of her companion's presence, the old maid from Manchester offering a homely lens through which to read and understand the 'other', with nineteenth-century ideas of femininity projected onto both.

Nevertheless, in case we might start to imagine that Head's description of the King Street museum is a progressive intervention centuries ahead of its time, he concludes his description by stating that, while the Egyptian damsel and the old maid were 'good of their sort', neither one 'was equal to the tattooed heads of New Zealand chiefs, now so commonly met with'.[20] Head offers no humanization or domestication of these 'tattooed heads', but simply expresses his excitement at seeing the newest fashion in displayed human remains.

* * *

As Head's account explained, the Manchester Natural History Society's collection outgrew its King Street premises in 1834, and the society took the decision to procure a new site for the museum. In 1835, after a decade of fundraising, the society was able to invest £4,000 in constructing a building on Peter Street that was substantially bigger than the rented King Street rooms.

The Peter Street museum was a purpose-built establishment, owned by the society, which stood close to the site of the 1819 Peterloo Massacre and a public hall that would host the Anti-Corn Law League in the late 1830s and early 1840s. Peter Street itself was relatively new, constructed in 1794 to facilitate a link between Quay Street (the quay on the River Irwell) and Mosley Street (the route to the city's commercial centre). The museum was situated just off Peter Street itself, on a side-street that came to be named Museum Street (a name it retains to this day, an occasional source of confusion for Mancunians, as there hasn't been a museum there since the late 1860s).

The new building had an entrance hall and two galleries on the ground floor, and a gallery and nine smaller rooms on the first floor. A sketch from 1865 shows a grand building with a two-storey pillared entrance. The institution opened its doors – though not to the public yet – on 18 May 1835. The man who had served as 'custodian' of the King Street museum, Timothy Harrop, was replaced by a new 'curator', William Crawford Williamson. Harrop was unflatteringly described by his successor as 'a man wholly ignorant of every branch of science except taxidermy, and he was probably the most accomplished bird-stuffer in Europe'.[21] By contrast, Williamson served as curator prior to completing his medical studies at University College, London, working as a doctor, and then embarking on an academic career after the formation of Owens College (later the Victoria University of Manchester). Williamson's interest in natural history had begun in his youth, as his father was a naturalist who was one of the first to explore the fossiliferous beds of the Yorkshire coast. By the time he was appointed curator of the society's museum, he had published papers on rare birds and fossils of Yorkshire, as well as a monograph on the Bronze Age 'Gristhorpe Man'.

Williamson's appointment was not without controversy, as he suggests in his memoirs:

> The greater and unscientific part of the council were in friendly sympathy with their old servant, but a few men of different stamp had recently been placed upon that council. These determined that what was then only a collection of ornamentally grouped birds should be made into a scientific museum, not only in the bird, but in all other departments.[22]

Despite resistance from the 'unscientific part of the council', and also the apparent readiness of Mancunians to exploit this unscientific nature and perpetrate hoaxes, including faking bird and fish specimens, Williamson spent his time as curator attempting to make 'a scientific museum'.[23]

Under Williamson's curation, the Peter Street museum retained the exclusivity of its former incarnation on King Street. Members of the society paid an annual subscription and an entrance fee if they wished to view the collection. On occasion, members were able to offer written invitations to friends who wished to 'inspect the treasures', but the wider population had no opportunity to do so.[24] Indeed, in 1837, the society's museum committee (the 'Governors') voted two to one against admitting the general public to the museum. At this time, all the other provincial society museums had adopted a policy of admitting fee-paying members of the public, and the Natural History Society's refusal to follow suit provoked criticism from Dr J. E. Gray of the British Museum, who 'commented unfavourably on the exclusiveness of the proprietors of the Manchester Museum'.[25]

In 1838, the decision to exclude the general public was revisited, and the museum's governors agreed to allow non-subscribers to visit the museum, on payment of a shilling (sixpence for the working classes, threepence for scholars). Shortly after this, Williamson was replaced as curator by Captain Thomas Brown and the museum entered into a new era of its existence.

Captain Brown was a military man, who became interested in natural history while quartered in Manchester with the Forfar and Kincardine Militia in 1813. By the time he took over from Williamson as curator, Brown had published illustrated books on conchology (shells) and lepidopterology (butterflies and moths), and he had also produced an edition of Oliver Goldsmith's *A History of the Earth and Illustrated Nature*, adding 'copious notes' and 'an appendix containing explanations of technical terms'.[26]

In the first year of Brown's curatorship, the museum welcomed 97 'Manchester' visitors (paying a shilling each), 1,286 'strangers' (also paying a shilling), 177 'Mechanics' (members of the Mechanics' Institute, or the respectable working class, paying sixpence each), 25 schoolchildren (paying sixpence each) and 14 'Sunday Scholars' (paying threepence each).[27] By the following year, this had risen to 1,681 visitors paying a shilling, 680 Mechanics, 42 schoolchildren and 1,353 Sunday Scholars.[28] In 1839, a guidebook to the city – *Manchester As It Is* – described the Peter Street museum as 'undoubtedly one of the most interesting Institutions of which the town can boast', noting that 'the ornithological collection stands the first in the provinces of Britain, if not Europe' and the entomological and conchological specimens are 'far from despicable' (which perhaps read as more complimentary in the 1830s). With good management, the guidebook suggests, this provincial museum 'might be made to rival some of the first metropolitan institutions'.[29]

It appears from the figures recorded in the annual reports of the Natural History Society's council that the decision to admit a wider audience was successful. It's easy to conclude that there was an appetite among certain strands of the public to 'inspect the treasures' of the society. The 'far from despicable' cabinet of insects was now on display to the general population of the city – mostly housed in 'British Room G' on the museum's first floor, along with shells and fish native to the British Isles.[30]

It may be imagined that, by throwing its doors open to the fee-paying public, the museum simply benefitted from a general appetite for natural history; however, the records of the society reveal a much more deliberate strategy on the part of the curator. In the Natural History Society's annual report of 1844, it's noted that:

> With the view of rendering the collection more useful, Captain Brown proposes giving a few gratuitous lectures, in the Museum, on Natural History, especially adapted for the young, during the Midsummer and Christmas holidays of the present year, to the Governors, Subscribers, and their families; in the course of which he will refer to the specimens for illustration of their character.[31]

While this early foray into a school holidays programme for the museum was limited to the families of governors and subscribers, it feels surprisingly close to modern museum practice. As I write this, the 2023 Midsummer holidays have begun, and the current Manchester Museum is offering 'Free Family Activities All Summer', including 'hands-on activities inspired by the objects and their stories'.[32]

But it was not just the young who were the target of Brown's innovative approach. By 1857, the society was taking bold, practical steps to encourage more working-class visitors into the museum:

> In the desire to make the Museum as much as possible a place of public resort, several Members of the Council made, during the summer months, great exertions to increase its attractions and instructive facilities. ... The Council, convinced by the experience of the past summer of the intelligent interest in the contents of the Museum, which is prevalent amongst the working classes, trust that their successors will prosecute to the utmost the measures they have adopted for making the opportunities afforded by the Society's Museum more widely known.[33]

This move to make the museum 'a place of public resort' included some proposed expenditure that is impressively perceptive: '[T]he

Council have had in consideration a project for lighting the Society's hall and rooms with gas, with a view to opening them to the public at the hours likely to be most welcome to the working classes.'[34] By 1863, the society were even considering the possibility of occasionally opening the museum for free:

> The attendance on the occasion of the Prince's marriage [Albert Edward, Prince of Wales, to Princess Alexandra of Denmark, in celebration of which the museum was open to the public for free, resulting more than six thousand visitors] shows what would be the popularity of the Museum if it could be thrown open to the general public free.[35]

It's exciting to think that the Natural History Society pre-empted Heritage Open Days by 131 years, and Museums at Night by 152 years, but this was possibly more a proactive response to the Museums Act 1845, to which we will return in a later chapter.

In 1857, the society's annual report noted that: 'No opportunity affords so effectual a means of elevating the tastes and pursuits of the working classes and young people of the district as frequent and intelligent resort to an extensive and, comparatively speaking, well-arranged Museum of Natural History, such as that of the Society.'[36] Nevertheless, not everybody agreed with this assessment of the museum's arrangement. As might be imagined, there was some tension between Captain Brown's drive to expand the visitor base for the museum and the society's role as a 'scientific museum'. In 1844, German travel writer Johan Georg Kohl published an account of his visit to the museum, in which, far from finding it 'well-arranged', he bemoaned the organization of the collections on display:

> I was displeased to find in this, so-called, Museum of Natural History, so many antiquarian relics, and ethnographical and historical remains, which, however interesting in themselves, had no business whatever here. This fault, however is not peculiar to the Museum of Manchester; it is more or less the defect of all the collections of Europe. This barbarous custom of spoiling different kinds of collections, by mixing them up together, without order or classification, has survived from those bygone times, in which scientific collections for definite purposes, were unknown, and when all kinds of 'curiosities' were esteemed equal and similar in value and importance. It is a piece of barbarism in science, thoroughly unworthy of this enlightened nineteenth century.[37]

The society's reports reveal a desire on the part of Captain Brown to make the collection 'useful' and a 'place of resort' for the general public. Kohl's complaint is that the museum should contain 'scientific collections for definite purposes' only. There is a hint here of the conflict between education and entertainment, between scholarship and inclusivity, which museums have yet to completely resolve to this day.

Under Captain Brown, the Peter Street museum became a public attraction, 'undoubtedly one of the most interesting Institutions of which the town can boast', with thousands of visitors passing through its doors to see its collection – 'barbarous' as it might have seemed to Kohl. In a retrospective assessment of the society's museum written in 1913, then President of the Manchester Lit and Phil, Francis Nicholson, suggested that: 'The general public were, it may be confessed, more interested in a few curiosities which owed their presence in the Museum to other circumstances than their value as specimens of Natural History.'[38] But we know already that this condescending view of the 'general public' who only went to the museum to see the 'curiosities' and didn't appreciate the 'valuable' specimens of natural history leaves out half the picture. George Head – the guest of a member of the academic society – reveals in his enthusiastic account that even the more scholarly guests of the King Street museum enjoyed its curiosities, including the preserved heads of New Zealand chiefs and the mummified bodies of an Egyptian damsel and a Mancunian old maid.

2

Behind the giraffe

When last we saw the Egyptian damsel and the Mancunian old maid, they were displayed together at the King Street museum, causing George Head to muse on a comparison between the 'ancient and modern art of embalming' and the 'services of the toilet' that made the two female corpses appear to be the same age. Both bodies were transferred to the Peter Street museum, and both were on display when the museum opened its doors to the wider public.

In 1839, a third mummy was introduced to the collection. The 'List of Donations' in the society's annual report for 1839 records the receipt of 'A Peruvian mummy, and relics picked up in the field of Waterloo, by Mr Stubbs, St Ann's-square'.[1] Little other information about this mummified body has survived, but it appears in various visitor accounts and society records from 1840.

In the previous chapter, we saw the criticisms of the museum's collection made by Johann Georg Kohl. Kohl visited the museum in the early 1840s and was displeased to find that, despite it being ostensibly a museum of natural history, specimens of the natural world were muddled up with 'antiquarian relics', 'ethnographical and historical remains' and 'all kinds of "curiosities"'.[2] However, although Kohl claimed that museum curiosities were 'thoroughly unworthy of this enlightened nineteenth century', his account goes on to reveal that he was actually quite taken with one particular 'curiosity':

> One of the most remarkable objects in the museum, is an English mummy, that of a Mrs Beswick, who gave orders in her testament that her body should not be buried, but should be embalmed, stuffed, and

> preserved by a certain Dr White, to whom, in reward, she bequeathed an annual income of 500*l*. On his death, the doctor bequeathed the body of the eccentric testatrix to the Museum of Manchester, where it now takes its place beside a Peruvian and Egyptian mummy.[3]

This is the earliest surviving origin story for the body that would come to be known as the 'Manchester Mummy', and it contains more information about the exhibit than is found in Head's account of his visit to the King Street museum just under a decade earlier.

Head was only able to furnish the information that the body was that of a 'lady of Manchester' who was 'old' and unmarried on her death, and to presume the method of preservation from the exhibit's visual appearance. By 1844, Kohl could supply a little more biographical detail, including the mummy's name, 'Mrs Beswick'. It's not clear from Kohl's account whether he is viewing the body of an 'old maid', as he gives the mummy the title 'Mrs'. This could well be an honorific based on her perceived age rather than her assumed marital status. What Kohl does give us is a clear and unequivocal assertion that the embalming of Mrs Beswick was carried out on an instruction left in the woman's will, and that 'a certain Dr White' was recompensed to the tune of £500 per year, though he offers no explanation as to *why* a woman – even an 'eccentric testatrix' – would wish to be 'embalmed, stuffed and preserved' on death, an experience that sounds more akin to taxidermy than to mummification.

We might also wonder why a doctor would acquiesce to such a request, as it hardly seems like appropriate behaviour for a medical professional. It's perhaps worth noting that in the 1830s (when the museum opened) and the 1840s (when Kohl had the opportunity to view the three mummies), public trust in the medical profession was at a distinct low. In considering the ways in which this distrust informed the popular imagination of the period, the literature scholar Joseph Crawford identifies 'four interlinked events: the Burke and Hare murders of 1828, the cholera epidemic of 1831–2, the Anatomy Act of 1832 and the New Poor Law of 1834'.[4]

Anatomists and surgeons had been associated with unsavoury practices of 'body-snatching' throughout the Georgian period – and not without reason. The transformation of surgery into an academic discipline created a pressing need for cadavers for demonstration purposes, and the more young men who wished to train as doctors, the more corpses were needed for the anatomy rooms.[5] By 1828, the issue was becoming a pressing one, with a parliamentary select committee drafting a 'Bill for preventing the unlawful disinterment of human bodies, and for regulating Schools of Anatomy', even before the murderous careers of William Burke and William Hare had come to light.

In her biography of anatomist, surgeon and midwife John Hunter, Wendy Moore outlines some of the techniques used by Georgian anatomists to procure bodies for their lecture theatres, including the bribing of 'unscrupulous undertakers to sell bodies prior to burial', leaving bereaved relatives to follow 'a coffin packed with stones in a funeral procession'.[6]

This scenario came true for one family in Manchester during the 1831–32 cholera epidemic. The high death toll during cholera outbreaks in the city led to panic, but it was the disposal of the bodies that caused real fear and anger among the working-class population of the city. Bodies were being buried in unconsecrated ground for expediency, and before the 1832 Anatomy Act was passed, the bodies of those who died in workhouses and prisons were given to doctors for the purposes of dissection. The case of Burke and Hare – men who are often described as 'body-snatchers' or 'resurrection men', stealing cadavers from fresh graves to sell to anatomists for dissection, but who actually murdered people to ensure a supply of bodies – was fresh in the mind, with 'burking' entering the vernacular as a verb meaning 'murder in order to sell the corpse for dissection'. The rapid burial of bodies in unconsecrated ground without observing funeral customs led people to believe that, in Crawford's words, 'doctors had something to hide: the fact that they had poisoned their patients, perhaps, or that they had stolen their bodies for dissection'.[7]

In late August 1832, John Brogan, the infant son of a weaver, died of cholera in Manchester. As his body was being buried, his grandfather, John Hayes, became suspicious when he noticed there was no name marked on the coffin lid. He interrupted the funeral and demanded that the coffin be opened. To his horror, he discovered his grandson's body had been decapitated, the head taken and replaced with a brick. John Hayes lived in Angel Meadow, a large industrial slum on the edge of Manchester, and author Dean Kirby includes an account of John Brogan's death and its aftermath in his book about this notorious part of the city. Kirby suggests that the panic that had been building during the epidemic reached 'boiling point' with the discovery of the mutilated body, resulting in the streets around Angel Meadow being 'engulfed in a vicious riot that dwarfed all those that had gone before'.[8] The assembled crowd – possibly as many as 3,000 people – surged towards Manchester's cholera hospital, shouting 'Pull it to the ground!'. The hospital was attacked, and four troops of hussars (the same regiment as had been sent into St Peter's Fields in what is now known as the Peterloo Massacre) were sent in to quell the riot. Eventually, it was discovered that the boy's body had been decapitated by a medical student named Robert Oldham, who had bribed a nurse to keep the secret.[9]

The cholera riot in Manchester – like others in urban districts around the country – was largely driven by the fear of the poorest residents of the city, fuelled by an awareness that it was terrifyingly easy for people of that class to find themselves in the workhouse or the prison and, thus, at the mercy of the anatomists. It could be argued that these people weren't the target market for the society's museum, which wouldn't offer reduced rates to working-class visitors until 1840, and then only to members of the Mechanics' Institute. Nevertheless, the fear of 'burking' wasn't limited to the working class. Astley Cooper, a member of the anatomical society formed in 1810 to lobby the government for legislation change, told the parliamentary select committee in 1828 that '[t]here is no person, let his situation in life be what it may, whom, if I were disposed to dissect, I could not obtain'.[10]

Evidence of the terror caused by resurrection men can still be discerned around the area now known as Greater Manchester. According to the memoirs of William Chadwick, a one-time Chief Constable of Stalybridge (around eight miles to the east of Manchester), the village of Cocker Hill was plagued by a group of body-snatchers in the early 1800s led by 'Captain Sellars', who would raid the graveyard after funerals to procure fresh corpses for sale.[11] It is still possible to see gravestones in Cocker Hill churchyard with the words 'This grave not to be reopened' carved into them. And a little further away, at St Michael and All Angels in Mottram-in-Longdendale, the grave of fifteen-year-old Lewis Brierley, who died in 1829, offers this chilling epitaph:

> Tho once beneath the ground his corpse was laid
> For use of surgeons it was thence convey'd.
> Vain was the scheme to hide the impious theft
> The body taken, shroud and coffin left.
> Ye wretches who pursue this barb'rous trade
> Your corpses in turn may be convey'd
> Like his to some unfeeling surgeons room
> Nor can they justly meet a better doom.

This is the context in which the unburied corpse of Miss Beswick – kept out of the grave by a doctor – was first exhibited in the centre of Manchester. For some, this might be considered proof that the medical profession really couldn't be trusted.

Of course, none of the early reports from visitors to the museum make any suggestion that Miss Beswick had been body-snatched, let alone burked, for the purposes of dissection. Indeed, Kohl's account is keen to point out that the preservation of the corpse was carried out at the request of the woman herself, and Head's flippant reference to the 'services of the toilet' carries the implication that the embalming of Asroni and Miss Beswick (one of whom undoubtedly was body-snatched, though Ancient Egyptian warnings that 'this grave is not to be reopened' have famously long been ignored) carried some benefits.

Nevertheless, both Head and Kohl offer some implicit criticism of the treatment of Miss Beswick's body. Head's use of the phrase 'the art of embalming' moves the practice away from funeral ritual and into the realms of display and exhibition, and Kohl's citation of the 'annual income of 500*l.*' received by Dr White attaches a slightly sordid monetary motive to the behaviour of the doctor.

The museum itself is unlikely to have encouraged a comparison of Miss Beswick's body with anti-medical hysteria and Gothic tales of resurrection men. The first curator of the Peter Street museum, William Crawford Williamson, was himself undertaking medical training. In his memoirs, Williamson refers to the practice of using cadavers in anatomy lectures, carefully noting that the Anatomy Act of 1832, passed as a result of both the cholera epidemics and the notoriety of the Burke and Hare case, ensured that the inmates of workhouses (though not prisons) were 'carefully protected'.[12]

As an aside, Williamson does somewhat undermine the gravity of his statement by following it with an anecdote to illustrate an unintended consequence of the Anatomy Act. After stating the provisions of the legislation, he continues:

> With each 'subject' arriving at the school, a coffin was sent to receive 'the remains' when they had served their purpose; which remains were forwarded for interment to a particular church, in one of the suburbs of Manchester. On one occasion, a lecturer had acquired a dead donkey, which was brought into our dissecting-room to be skeletonised for its owner. When this was accomplished, all other 'remains' of the animal were put, by some of the mischief-loving students, into one of the vacant coffins, and the coffin sent as usual to church for interment; the mischievous young monkeys attending in order to witness the clergyman perform the solemn service of burial over his 'dear departed brother'.[13]

When read alongside Kirby's account of the cholera riots, and his description of the work of Father Daniel Hearne (Catholic) and Reverend John Smith (Wesleyan) to ensure the decent burial of cholera victims in churches in the suburbs of Manchester, including retrieving the head of young John Brogan from the lodgings of a medical student, sewing it back onto the child's body, and conducting a solemn service of burial at St Patrick's Church, Williamson's tale of the 'mischievous young monkeys' in the late 1830s seems a wee bit distasteful.[14]

That said, Williamson's intention is to present dissection for the purposes of anatomical study as a necessary and regulated practice for the medical profession. The Manchester Lit and Phil – and likely by association the Manchester Natural History Society – had a significant relationship with the personnel (physicians and trustees) of the town's infirmary.[15] Given that a number of members of the Natural History Society had similar medical or academic training to Williamson, their experience and opinion of the medical profession is likely to have differed dramatically from that of the residents of Angel Meadow, and their interpretation of the actions of Dr White on the body of Miss Beswick may have had a particular bias.

However, once the museum was opened to a wider viewing public – the friends of subscribers who attended the King Street museum, or the general public who visited the Peter Street museum – the society no longer had control of the narrative. While they could provide information about the artefacts on display, each visitor brought their own assumptions and perspectives through which they would view the exhibits. Additionally, while I make no suggestion that the museum or the society deliberately fostered a mistrust of Dr White or his motives in their display of the body of Miss Beswick, the curatorial practices did little to dispel potential suspicion.

* * *

No formal catalogue was ever produced for the Peter Street museum, and later accounts suggest that the information given about exhibits within the display cases was minimal at best. Writers and scholars who have attempted to study the museum in the years following its closure – myself included – have found themselves frustrated by poor-to-non-existent recordkeeping, and a somewhat cavalier attitude towards recording both the provenance and acquisition details of certain items in the collection. For example, Francis Nicholson, writing about the museum in 1913, noted that 'no complete catalogue of the Museum was ever issued, and the manuscript lists were very brief'.[16]

The Peter Street museum was not – and is not – unique in this failing. I've already mentioned the Peruvian mummy donated to the museum in 1839. Outside of the reference to Mr Stubbs donating the mummy, there is no further information about the provenance given, nor any record of information pertaining to its age, sex or location of discovery. All that remains of its existence as an exhibit are details of valuations made of the museum's collections in 1845 and 1849, which list the value of the 'Peruvian Mummy and Case' at £10, the same value ascribed to the 'Mummy of Miss Beswick' but substantially less than the 'Egyptian Mummy with Case and Sarcophigi [*sic*]' (£100) and the 'Skeleton of Elephant' (£80).[17]

Although the museum never produced a complete catalogue of its exhibitions, an attempt *was* made to record and describe the collection for the public. In 1856, Thomas Ashton, a Manchester doctor, documented the museum's collections for a publication entitled *Visits to the Museum of the Manchester Natural History Society*, which was published by the society itself. Ashton's preface to the volume states that he has been asked to produce 'a brief account of the contents of the Museum' that is 'intended merely for popular use'.[18] He states that a partial account, describing only a portion of the museum's collection, had already sold 2,000 copies before the full version was completed. The first edition of Ashton's *Visits* was published in 1857, followed by further editions in 1860 and 1863.

Ashton's *Visits* is invaluable to understanding the Peter Street museum, and not only because it is the closest thing to a catalogue you can get. As the book was intended for a general, rather than scholarly, audience, Ashton captures something of the experience of walking around the museum, allowing the reader (even in the twenty-first century) to conjure an image of the Peter Street premises in their mind. Indeed, as he 'travels' through the museum room by room, it is the first – and only – account that allows a reader to really imagine what the Peter Street museum was like.

Using Ashton's *Visits* as a guide, we enter Room B, to the right of the entrance hall on the ground floor, and come face-to-face with the 'New Zealander's head' (which George Head had admired over twenty years earlier). Ashton gives us no indication of the history of the object, but merely offers a little light background on the practice of facial tattooing among the 'islanders'. In the same room of 'Curiosities', we can find 'Peruvian Mummy' (which, we learn, is 'merely dipped in bitumen and buried in a sack in sand') and 'Sarcophagi' belonging to 'the Egyptian mummy extended here'. This latter exhibit has some backstory: 'This mummy, embalmed upwards of 2,900 years since, is the body of Asroni, a maid of honour in the court of the 20th Pharaoh, and daughter of Phasco, scribe, of Lower Egypt.' Ashton goes on to offer clarification:

> Properly speaking, mummy is not the body, but the composition used for its preservation. Bitumen or asphaltum is supposed to have been anciently used, but odipherous substances were also employed, and the cost of embalming varied from a very small sum to a talent of silver, about £300.[19]

The two ancient mummies are thus exhibited together as 'Curiosities', as they had been when Kohl visited in 1844, but their Mancunian companion is now absent. We might look around the other curiosities in Room B, taking in 'Horns of Narwhals or Sea Unicorns', a 'Model of the Valley of the Irwell', a 'Large Burmese Idol' and a 'Stuffed Shark', but we won't see the body of Miss Beswick.[20]

And that's because we missed her when we arrived. Ashton's account starts with Room A (to the left of the Entrance Hall) and Room B (to the right) before returning us to the Entrance Hall itself. And here, we will see curiosities indeed.

There is a stuffed giraffe ('the tallest, though not the bulkiest of all animals') and an elephant ('with a trunk of the most extraordinary qualities'). There is also the '[s]kull of a horse, Old Billy, which attained the great age of 62 years, the oldest on record but one, which lived to 72. Billy belonged to the Mersey and Irwell Navigation Company'. And then, we are told:

> In a case behind the giraffe is a mummy more curious for its history than from any peculiarity in itself. It is the body of *Miss Beswick*, once an affluent Manchester lady, a relative of whom having been buried in a swoon, as was supposed, was never afterwards free from the dread of being interred alive. She therefore bequeathed to her medical advisor a property of considerable value which he was to enjoy 'so long as he kept her above ground'. By process of mummifying, the body was preserved in a case during his life, and the intent of both parties has been fulfilled.[21]

Ashton's 'Miss Beswick' bears some comparison with Kohl's 'Mrs Beswick' of 1844. Both descriptions underline the woman's wealth, and both assert that the mummification was carried out on the woman's express instruction.

There are, however, clear differences between the two accounts. While Kohl attributes the woman's final wishes simply to her being an 'eccentric testatrix', Ashton ascribes it to pathological taphophobia (the fear of being buried alive), making the actions of her 'medical advisor' a merciful, rather than a mercenary, act. He even goes so far as to offer what appears to be a quote from the woman's will, clearly stating her desire to have her remains kept 'above ground'. Interestingly, while Kohl names Miss Beswick's doctor, Ashton does not, and this is a very curious detail. As a medical doctor himself, Thomas Ashton could have been in no doubt as to who 'Dr White' actually was.

It is possible that Ashton was unfamiliar with Kohl's earlier account of a visit to the museum. This would explain why, in 1844, a visitor was advised that the woman was embalmed by 'Dr White', but by 1856 this information had either been forgotten or not passed on when Ashton visited the museum. Or, perhaps, Ashton decided not to name Dr White out of professional respect. It's impossible to know for sure, but the discrepancy certainly suggests that there was no 'official' story about the mummy on display in the museum, and that visitors pieced together their own narrative based partly on what they were told, and partly on their own preconceptions.

Of course, it's the fear of premature burial that's the most significant detail of Ashton's account. This detail remains part of the Manchester Mummy story to this day, and various popular accounts of the case replicate this detail without question – though often with a degree of embellishment.

By the time Ashton wrote his account, the fear of burking and body-snatching had receded in the popular imagination. In popular fiction, the figure of the 'resurrection man' reached its zenith with the 1844–45 publication of *The Mysteries of London*, a Gothic penny publication by George W. M. Reynolds. This penny blood, which featured a villain known as the Resurrection Man, who is both a body-snatcher and a murderer, was one of the most widely read pieces of fiction of the early Victorian period and was enthusiastically sold for Mancunian readers at Abel Heywood's bookshop on Oldham Street (a relatively short walk from Peter Street).[22] After this, the fictional body-snatcher wouldn't be resurrected with any zeal until Robert Louis Stephenson's short story 'The Body Snatcher' was published in 1884. By the time the first series of *The Mysteries of London* came to an end, not only had the fashion for villainous, murdering grave-robbers come to an end in popular culture, the actual practice of body-snatching had almost entirely died out in England, with only one reported case taking place after 1844.

In addition to this, the setting up of local boards of health and municipal borough corporations – the local authorities formed in urban areas to address health and sanitation concerns following the cholera epidemics – had shifted the focus of public health anxieties from doctors, hospitals and medical schools to municipal authorities. Manchester Council and its associated corporation came into existence in 1838, though the town had seen local governance of a more embryonic form prior to this, with civic administration operating first from the police offices and then from a purpose-built town hall on King Street in 1825. When the town was incorporated in 1838, the town hall on King Street became the premises of the Manchester Corporation (and, later, the elected Town Council) and the place where decisions about public health would now be taken by elected representatives of (some of) the people. The sinister doctor misusing stolen corpses belonged to the penny fiction of previous decades, rather than the brave new municipal world of Victorian Manchester.

Taphophobia is pretty much the opposite of body-snatching. The latter is the body being taken from the grave after death, while the former is a fear of being placed into the grave while still alive. However, it still evokes a certain distrust of the medical profession and its practitioners. In *Buried Alive,* his extensive study of what he calls 'our most primal fear', Jan Bondeson catalogues numerous cases of apparent 'premature burial', the majority of which involve an inobservant or incompetent medical attendant pronouncing death when it has not actually occurred.[23] As Bondeson argues, this may well have been a result of changing scientific and medical knowledge around signs of death and signs of life in a supposed corpse. It may also have been an indication of anxieties around changes in funeral practice and the accepted means of disposing of bodies.

The idea of the 'premature burial' surfaces in the popular imagination at particular points in time, and the mid-nineteenth century is one of those points. Fiction – most famously Edgar Allan Poe's short story 'The Premature Burial' (1844) – revelled in the macabre possibilities of being buried alive, but Bondeson argues that Poe would have had 'background reading' on the subject from periodicals at the time. He states:

> In the 1830s and 1840s, it was neither uncommon nor abnormal to be concerned about the risk of being buried alive; indeed, some of the

> leading European medical authorities on the subject were of the opinion that live burials were common. The popular newspapers and magazines, like *Blackwood's Edinburgh Magazine*, the *Casket*, the *Southern Literary Messenger*, and the *New-York Mirror*, frequently published stories of premature interment – some of them plainly fictional, others claiming a factual origin.[24]

The final sentence of this quote reveals the problem with considerations of taphophobia – it is almost impossible to differentiate between fictional accounts and factual ones, meaning it's very hard to say how many people have genuinely been worried about premature burial as a real possibility, versus how many people have just enjoyed reading about it in gleefully Gothic and occasionally gory prose.

Bondeson himself falls into this trap in his otherwise rigorous and well-researched study, including at least two accounts that are presented as factual evidence for the phobia, when the reality is a little less secure. The first is his assertion that, in 1852, a man named George Bateson acquired a patent for the Bateson Life Revival Device (known as the 'Belfry'), a 'security coffin' with 'an iron bell mounted in a miniature campanile on the lid of the casket'. Bondeson goes on to give a potted history of Bateson's career – including an OBE from Queen Victoria for 'services to the dead' – and personal anxieties around burial – culminating in his self-immolation to avoid being buried alive.[25] But, as Jeremy Stern revealed, in a 2013 article for the *History News Network* website of the Columbian College of Arts and Sciences, George Bateson and the Life Revival Device never actually existed. The whole story was invented by the novelist Michael Crichton for his 1975 book *The Great Train Robbery*; however, an article in a medical journal in 1975 cited his description of Bateson's Belfry as a historical account, and it is this citation – alongside the reference to Crichton's novel – that is included in the endnotes of Bondeson's book.[26] Now, any study of premature burial that wishes to list a 'verified' example of a patented 'security coffin' can include Bateson's Belfry and cite Bondeson's book as the source.

This type of self-fulfilling reference can also be found in the second of the examples in the book: Bondeson's inclusion of the story of Miss Beswick as evidence of eighteenth-century concerns about being buried alive. Bondeson presents the story of Miss Beswick, complete with pathological taphophobia, the brother's narrow escape, and the bequest to her doctor to ensure her body 'never be buried', as historical fact.[27] The endnotes give three sources to back these claims up: a 1966 article in *Medicolegal Journal*, which turns out to include the story of Miss Beswick but without any sources, a 1994 article in *Udolpho*, the magazine of the Gothic Society, and Edith Sitwell's 1933 book *The English Eccentrics*, which contains absolutely no footnotes or evidence for its claims but does inexplicably note that Miss Beswick had 'thick black eyebrows' when she died.[28] Nevertheless, any study of premature burial that now wishes to include Miss Beswick as a 'real life' example of taphophobia can do so, citing Bondeson's book itself as the source.

It's clear that the *idea* of premature burial has existed in the popular imagination for a long time, and that it is deeply rooted in anxieties about the medical profession, funeral practice and the scientific understanding of death and dying. The problem revealed in Bondeson's study is that it is very difficult to differentiate fictional accounts from those with a factual origin, meaning it is very hard, in the absence of primary sources, to conclusively prove that an individual took practical steps to avoid this fate in the event of their demise.

In writing his brief account of the mummy of Miss Beswick, Thomas Ashton sets in stone one of the key 'facts' that will become almost canonical in later versions of the story: she was terrified of being buried alive and took practical steps to prevent this from occurring. Ashton offers no proof for this assertion, and the story is decidedly vague and lacking in detail, such as when or where it happened. However, the idea that pathological taphophobia is a genuine fear, and that it is evidenced by idiosyncratic burial practices, is so real in the popular imagination that Ashton's story has been taken at face value ever since it first appeared in print.

* * *

Four years before Ashton published the first edition of his *Visits*, a quite different book was published by a writer who, though originally a native of Manchester, likely never visited the Peter Street museum. And yet, it has undeniable significance to the story.

Thomas de Quincey was born in Manchester in 1785. He is perhaps best known now for his work *Confessions of an English Opium-Eater* (published in 1821), but he was also an essayist, journalist, critic and translator who published a large collection of writing during his lifetime. In 1853–54, shortly before de Quincey's death, a collection of his writings appeared under the title *Autobiographic Sketches*, and in this work he writes about his friendship with a doctor he calls 'Mr White'.

A previous work, *Suspiria de profundis* (1845), had mentioned 'Mr White' as a surgeon called in to assist with the illness of de Quincey's sister Elizabeth in 1792. 'Mr White', as becomes apparent in de Quincey's later writings, is Charles White (1728–1813), a surgeon and midwife who was one of the founders of both the Manchester Infirmary (later the Manchester Royal Infirmary) and the Lying-In Hospital (later St Mary's Hospital). In *Autobiographic Sketches*, de Quincey elaborates on his relationship with Charles White, noting that the doctor befriended him when he was a teenager. After the death of his father in 1793, his mother moved to Bath, and de Quincey attended schools in Somerset and Wiltshire. When he was fifteen, he was sent back to Manchester to attend Manchester Grammar School and it was here, as a lonely and apparently miserable young man, that Charles White took him under his wing. In *Autobiographic Sketches*, de Quincey offers a brief introduction to the career and personality of the doctor:

> Mr White, whom I have already had occasion to mention, was in those days the most eminent surgeon by much in the North of England. He had by one whole generation run before the phrenologists and craniologists – having already measured innumerable skulls amongst the omnigenous seafaring population of Liverpool, illustrating all the races of men; and was in society a most urbane and pleasant companion.[29]

He then goes on to recount an episode that took place during this period of 'intimacy' during de Quincey's brief return to Manchester:

> Mr White possessed a museum – formed chiefly by himself, and originally, perhaps, directed simply to professional objects, such as would have little chance for engaging the attention of females. But surgeons and speculative physicians, beyond all other classes of intellectual men, cultivate the most enlarged and liberal curiosity; so that Mr White's museum furnished attractions to an unusually large variety of tastes. I had myself already seen it[.]

de Quincey then explains that he has forgotten everything about the objects 'which gave a scientific interest to the collection', recalling only the curiosities, the human remains. He states that Mr White had two significant exhibits in his collection, a skeleton and 'a mummy'. To his dismay, when he takes his friend Lady Carbery to see the museum, during the episode he is recounting, only the skeleton was on display. This leads to the following explanation:

> Perhaps the mummy was too closely connected with the personal history of Mr White for exhibition to strangers! it was that of a lady who had been attended medically for some years by Mr White, and had owed much alleviation of her sufferings to his inventive skill. She had therefore felt herself called upon to memorialize her gratitude by a very large bequest, not less (I have heard) than £25,000; but with this condition annexed to the gift – that she should be embalmed as perfectly as the resources in that art of London and Paris could accomplish, and that once a year Mr White, accompanied by two witnesses of credit, should withdraw the veil from her face. The lady was placed in a common English clock-case, having the usual glass face: but a veil of white velvet obscured from all profane eyes the silent features behind. The clock I had myself seen, when a child, and had gazed upon it with inexpressible awe. But naturally, on my report of the case, the whole of our party were devoured by a curiosity to see the departed fair one. Had Mr White, indeed, furnished us with the key of the museum, leaving us to our own discretion, but restricting us only (like a cruel Bluebeard) from looking into any ante-room, great is my fear that the perfidious question would have arisen amongst us – what o'clock it was? and all possible anterooms would have given way to the just fury of our passions. [...] Thus, however, it happened that the mummy, who left such valuable legacies, and founded such bilious fevers of curiosity, was not seen by us; nor even the miserable clock-case.[30]

What to make of de Quincey's account of Mr White's museum? Is this a description of the 'old maid' in the Peter Street museum?

Thomas de Quincey's mummy isn't given a name, though she is clearly a very wealthy woman. As in Kohl and Ashton's accounts, she is an 'eccentric testatrix' on whose instructions the embalming is carried out. There is, again as in Kohl and Ashton's accounts, a large monetary reward for the doctor in return for his unorthodox post-mortem services, and there is also the placement of the body in a museum, though this appears to be the private cabinet of a medical doctor for 'professional' demonstrations rather than 'exhibition to strangers'. It may also be remembered that Kohl asserted that the doctor who embalmed the mummy in the Peter Street museum had embalmed her some time prior to the museum's creation, and the body was the bequeathed to the museum on the death of the doctor, which does fit with de Quincey's testimony.

Nevertheless, there are some marked differences between de Quincey's account and those of the visitors to the Peter Street museum. The stipulation that Dr White must inspect the body's face once a year in the presence of witnesses is a detail that doesn't appear in the accounts of the Peter Street 'old maid', and the nature of the bequest is also substantially different to the other versions of the story. de Quincey also doesn't name the mummy, noting simply that she was a patient of White's in her lifetime.

There are also some strange discrepancies within de Quincey's account itself. Firstly, it isn't completely apparent whether the author has actually laid eyes on the mummy itself. He begins by stating that he has previously seen the museum, and by his enthusiastic endorsement of its 'humanities', particularly the mummy in the clock case, we might easily assume that he has personally viewed that particular exhibit. However, later in his account, he says that he had seen the clock case when he was a child, implying that he hadn't actually seen the mummy inside it.

Furthermore, de Quincey's account of the woman's instructions and legacy hold very little water. He claims that the woman stipulated that she wanted to be embalmed 'as perfectly as the resources in that art of London and Paris could accomplish' with White inspecting his handiwork once a year, but no explanation for this utterly bizarre request is given. The bequest she allegedly makes to White is also deeply suspect. The sum of £25,000 is a remarkable amount of money, roughly the equivalent of £4,000,000 today, which surely would've been life-altering, even for a wealthy and eminent surgeon.

In his consideration of de Quincey's account of his interactions with Dr White, Peter Kitson describes his writing as 'baroque', suggesting that de Quincey became 'almost fixated with White' after a 'primal scene of his childhood', when he watched White and his colleague

Thomas Percival attend to the death of his sister Elizabeth.[31] There are certainly elements in the description of Dr White's museum that might lead to this conclusion, for instance the flight-of-fancy as to what might have happened if the doctor had, 'like a cruel Bluebeard', allowed his visitors access to all rooms except the one housing the mummy.

Regardless of the reliability of de Quincey's account, the description of Charles White's museum, including the mummy in the clock case, doesn't seem to have had any impact on the presentation of the mummy in the Peter Street museum. The second and third editions of Ashton's *Visits* were published in 1860 and 1863 with no amendments made to the information given about Miss Beswick. As noted earlier, it may be that Ashton – who, as a Manchester doctor, could not have been unfamiliar with the work of Charles White, a man who not only founded two of the most significant medical establishments in the city, but also published frequently cited textbooks and gave lectures at the Manchester Lit and Phil on the subject of anatomy – resisted naming Dr White in his account out of professional courtesy. Or, of course, it may simply be that Ashton never read de Quincey's *Autobiographic Sketches* and so was never aware of this account of the mummy's former habitation in the private collection of the doctor who embalmed her.

3

The ungenteel fate

In 1797, the French geologist and travel writer Barthélemy Faujas de Saint-Fond published *Voyage en Angleterre, en Écosse et aux Îles Hébrides*, which recounted a trip taken around England, Scotland and the Hebrides. During this trip, Faujas de Saint-Fond paid a visit to the London home of Dr John Sheldon, an anatomist and surgeon who, according to the author, possessed 'one of the finest anatomical cabinets in existence'.[1] After spending some time talking with Sheldon about their shared love of hot air balloons, Faujas de Saint-Fond devoted several mornings to visiting Sheldon's anatomical cabinet and exploring the preparations collected by its owner. He comments on some interesting illustrations in the collection, before adding – in a turn of phrase that should come as no surprise at this point in our story – 'but nothing in this collection interested so much as a kind of mummy'.[2]

That said, what follows may come as a surprise, and not in a good way:

> I was introduced into a very handsome bed-room; a mahogany table of an oblong form, stood in the midst of it, facing the bed.
>
> The top of this table opened by a groove, and under a glass-frame I saw the body of a young woman, of nineteen or twenty, entirely naked. She had fine brown hair, and lay extended as on a bed.
>
> The glass was lifted up, and Sheldon made me admire the flexibility of the arms, a kind of elasticity in the bosom, and even in the cheeks, and the perfect preservation of the other parts of the body. Even the skin partly retained its colour, though exposed to the air.

> It appeared to me, however, that the fleshy parts were rather dry, and that there was too great a tenseness of the muscles. This gave to the figure, though it still possessed the remains of beauty, a meagre and feeble air, which considerably diminished the delicacy of its traits.[3]

Sheldon then outlines the method he used to prepare his mummy, which Faujas de Saint-Fond relates in full before asking the obvious question: *why?*

> He replied frankly, and without any hesitation, 'It is a mistress whom I tenderly loved. I paid every attention to her during a long sickness, and a short time before her death, she requested that I should make a mummy of her body, and keep her beside me – I have kept my word to her.'[4]

Faujas de Saint-Fond muses on the implications of this, relating it to what he knows of Egyptian mummification practices. He expresses some distaste for what his friend has done, but quickly reminds himself and his readers that Sheldon is 'gentle and compassionate' and concludes: 'Let us quit, however, this dismal subject, and proceed to describe the dinner which I had with some of the members of the Royal Society.'[5] Meanwhile, in another part of London, a corpse was displayed in the front room of dentist's home surgery.

Maria van Butchell (formerly Mary Billion) died in 1775, and her husband Martin van Butchell paid to have her embalmed by the eminent surgeon, anatomist and midwife William Hunter. van Butchell then displayed the body of his dead wife, along with the taxidermized body of her pet parrot, for patrons of his surgery to see. The body was such a popular curiosity that van Butchell was forced to place an advertisement in the newspaper: 'Van Butchell (not willing to be unpleasantly circumstanced and wishing to convince some good minds that they have been misinformed) acquaints the Curious, no stranger can see his embalmed wife, unless (by a Friend personally) introduced to himself, any day between Nine and One, Sundays excepted.'[6]

In 1808, John Sheldon's widow presented his mummy, which had by then acquired the name 'Miss Johnson', to the Hunterian Museum in London, where it was displayed with the description:

> The embalmed body of a female subject aged 24, of the name of Johnson, who died of phthisis in the Lock Hospital, about the year 1775 and left

> her body for dissection to Mr Sheldon, who was at that time a pupil of that charity [...] Presented by Mrs Rebecca Sheldon Dec 24th 1808.[7]

And in 1815, the late Martin van Butchell's son donated the embalmed body of Maria van Butchell to the Hunterian Museum, where it was put on display next to the body of Miss Johnson. The two mummies were exhibited side by side in the museum until 1941, when the building was hit by a bomb and the bodies were both destroyed.

In the same year as Maria van Butchell's body was donated to the Hunterian Museum, Saartje (Sarah) Baartman died. A Khoikhoi woman from southwestern Africa, Baartman was taken from her homeland to Europe by surgeon Alexander Dunlop to be exhibited at fairs, shows and private parties. From 1810 until her death in 1815, she was exhibited around various locations in Europe as the 'Hottentot Venus', a sexualized and dehumanized living curiosity.[8] She was in Manchester in 1811, when *The Times* described her as 'the African fair one who has so greatly attracted the notice of the town'.[9]

When Baartman died, her remains were dissected and preserved by Frédéric Cuvier, a zoologist, palaeontologist and keeper of the menagerie at the Muséum d'Histoire Naturelle in Paris, who then had them displayed in the Muséum d'Histoire Naturelle d'Angers. The remains were moved to the Musée de l'Homme in 1937, where her skeleton and a full body cast remained until the 1970s, turned to the side to emphasis the steatopygia (fat and tissue on the buttocks and thighs) that was the 'unique selling point', and object of sexualized fascination, for Baartman in both life and death.

In the year George Head visited the King Street museum in Manchester to wax lyrical about the body of Miss Beswick, a woman named Julia Pastrana was born in Mexico. Pastrana was an indigenous woman who suffered from hypertrichosis (abnormal hair growth). There are conflicting and unverified accounts of Pastrana's early life, but by 1854, when she was around twenty years old, she was 'performing' or being exhibited in freak shows and fairs in the United States. She married Theodore Lent in 1855, who took over the management of Pastrana's 'act'. She was toured around the United States and Europe as, among other names, 'Baboon Lady', 'Dog-faced Woman', 'Ape Woman' and 'The Nondescript'.

After her death, Pastrana's husband sold her body and the body of their infant son (who died three days after his birth, leading to Pastrana's death from post-birth complications) to be taxidermically preserved by a Professor Sukolov of Moscow University, who then sold them back to Theodore Lent to be exhibited at fairs, museums and amusement parks. The bodies of Pastrana and her infant son were exhibited until the 1970s, before being withdrawn from public display in 1972 and ending up in the Department of Anatomy at Oslo University.

The remains of Saartje Baartman and Julia Pastrana are no longer on display or held in museum collections. After decades of campaigning for the repatriation of her remains – including a formal request by President Nelson Mandela in 1994 – Baartman was buried in Hankey in the Eastern Cape on 9 August 2002. The municipal district which includes Hankey is now known as the Sarah Baartman District. And in 2012, after a campaign led by, among others, artist Laura Anderson Barbata, the remains of Julia Pastrana were turned over to authorities in Sinaloa, Mexico, and then buried with a Catholic funeral service in Sinaloa de Leyva in February 2013.

But, for a time, it was possible to see the bodies of all of these women – Miss Beswick, Miss Johnson, Maria van Butchell, Saartje Baartman and Julia Pastrana – on display in Manchester, London, Paris and various other locations around Europe, as indeed many people did.

* * *

These were not the only preserved dead bodies that you could view at the time. Miss Johnson and Maria van Butchell were displayed alongside three Egyptian mummies, a Peruvian mummy and a 'Guanche, or mummy, from the ancient sepulchres in the island of Teneriffe'.[10] As noted in a previous chapter, the body of Miss Beswick was exhibited in Manchester alongside the Egyptian mummy known as Asroni and an unnamed Peruvian mummy.

While we don't have any details about the Peruvian mummy displayed in Manchester, a contemporaneous (*c.* 1830s–40s) flyer advertising an exhibit in Rochester gives us some context. This 'extraordinary Peruvian relic' was 'the entire body of a Peruvian woman, perfect as when in life' and was to be exhibited at a private premises in Rochester, admission sixpence. The advertisement explains that the 'unparalleled curiosity' was taken from its burial place 'about 100 miles from Arica' by a Captain Woods, who was exploring the region on horseback:

> This PERUVIAN RELIC is the entire body of a female, who is supposed to have been buried alive several hundred years ago. The body being exhumed, it was found to be in a state of the most PERFECT PRESERVATION, although bearing indubitable evidence that it must have been interred at a remote period of time.[11]

It goes on:

> The features are perfect and convey a distinct idea of what they were when animated. The hair on the head is abundant, and finely preserved, being ingeniously plaited over the shoulders, it seems to have been originally black but has been changed into an amber hue, probably by the action of the sun. The eye-brows and eye lashes are perfect, the teeth firm in their places, the finger and toes nails entire, the skin whole and the flesh firm and dry. [...] There is nothing unpleasant or offensive in the appearance of this curious Relic; producing only sympathy and regret for the dreadful fate of the unhappy victim of Peruvian barbarity, and may be seen without the slightest insult to decency or modesty.

As I've previously noted, Angela Stienne's exploration of the stories behind Egyptian mummies held in museum collections identifies an 'insidious political message', one that that carries both racial and cultural weight, that is conveyed through the exhibition and viewing of the bodies (dead and alive) of 'real people'.[12]

It is impossible not to read such an 'insidious political message' in the presentation of the 'Hottentot Venus' and 'The Nondescript', women who (in life and in death) were viewed through the lens of colonialism, white superiority and polygenism (the scientific theory that different races were, in fact, different species). We can also see evidence of it in the advertisement for the Peruvian mummy in Rochester, which promises the viewer (assumed white and British) will feel 'sympathy and regret for the dreadful fate of the unhappy victim of Peruvian barbarity', and – earlier in the description – offers the explanation that

Captain Woods was in danger of 'falling a sacrifice to the resentment of the natives' when he retrieved the body.[13]

Miss Johnson and Maria van Butchell were, it is assumed, white European women, residents (if not natives) of London. And yet, we can see a process of othering in their presentation that bears some comparison with that of Saartje Baartman, Julia Pastrana and the unnamed Peruvian woman in Rochester. Firstly, there is a rather obsessive attention to details of traditionally feminine physical features in the descriptions of the women's corpses. Miss Johnson is described in terms of her arms, bosom and the 'remains of beauty', just as the Peruvian mummy has abundant plaited hair and perfect brows and lashes. Saartje Baartman is a 'Venus', known (and imitated) for the shape of her buttocks. In the case of Baartman, these details become explicitly sexualized. In the case of Miss Johnson, the sexualization is implicit but nevertheless just as permanent: there are few accounts of Miss Johnson's story that don't include the claim made by Sheldon's widow that the woman was a patient in the Lock Hospital. The London Lock Hospital was an institution founded to treat venereal disease, specifically syphilis, so every time the body is linked to the hospital (even innocently) the spectre of sexually transmitted disease is raised.

In addition to this, accounts reveal a fascination with the lifelike quality of these preserved corpses, which is juxtaposed with the sharp reminders of death. The Peruvian mummy is 'perfect as when in life', as Miss Johnson has skin that 'partly retained its colour'; but the former is 'firm and dry', and the latter is 'rather dry' with 'a tenseness of the muscles'. An advertisement for an exhibition of Julia Pastrana's corpse in Piccadilly in 1862 (admission 2s. 6d.) refers to the body as 'the exact life-like specimen of embalming', and goes on to present testimony from a F. T. Buckland, who apparently had seen the woman displayed in both life and death:

> The figure is dressed in the ordinary exhibition costume used in life, and is placed erect upon a table. The limbs are by no means shrunken or contracted, the arms, chest, &c. retaining their former roundness and well-formed appearance. The face is marvellous; it is exactly like an exceedingly good portrait in wax, but it *not* formed of wax. The closest examination convinced me that it was the true skin, prepared in

> some wonderful way; the huge deformed lips and the squat nose remain exactly as in life; and the beard and luxuriant growth of soft black hair on and about the face are in no respect changed from their former appearance. There is no unpleasant odour, or other disagreeable concomitant, about the figure; it is almost difficult to imagine that it is really that of a human being, and not an artificial model.[14]

Pastrana's body is both lifelike and unlifelike, animate and inanimate. The vestiges of her feminine form are enthused over, with even her 'monstrous' qualities – the 'deformed lips', 'squat nose' and 'beard' – transformed into a fantasy of luxuriance and sensuality. The reassurance that there is 'no unpleasant odour' is our subtle reminder that the exhibit being described is actually a dead body.

* * *

Another similarity between the descriptions of the preserved corpses under consideration in this chapter is the persistent suggestion that the mummification or preservation of the body after death was, at least in part, a desire expressed when the woman was alive. Faujas de Saint-Fond's account of viewing Miss Johnson's corpse includes supposed testimony from John Sheldon that 'a short time before her death, she requested that I should make a mummy of her body, and keep her beside me', and the information provided by Rebecca Sheldon when the mummy was deposited with the Hunterian Museum was that she 'left her body for dissection to Mr Sheldon'.

The idea that the displayed female corpse may actually be the realization of a woman's wishes takes on an added dimension in the cases of Saartje Baartman and Julia Pastrana, women who were exhibited in life as well as in death.

Shortly after the passing of the 1807 Slave Trade Act, Baartman was taken to London to be exhibited by Hendrik Cesars. Abolitionist Zachary Macaulay and the Association for Promoting the Discovery of the Interior Parts of Africa (also known as the Africa Association) took Cesars to court, arguing that Baartman was an enslaved person and should be released. William Bullock of Liverpool Museum gave testimony in support of the prosecution, stating that Baartman was referred to as a piece of property by the men who brought her to Britain. In his defence,

Cesars argued that Baartman was 'performing' by her own freely given consent, asking 'has she not as good a right to exhibit herself as an Irish Giant or a Dwarf?'[15] Baartman, speaking through a Dutch interpreter, gave testimony that she was not under restraint, performed of her own volition and was recompensed for her performances.

Pastrana's case offers a similar implication of free will, though without the associated legal proceedings. Although accounts suggest that the young Pastrana was indeed bought like a piece of property, an article in the *Baltimore Sun* in 1855 described how she escaped her captivity to 'elope' with Theodore Lent, becoming a willing participant in a showbusiness partnership.[16]

Although neither case involves any direct assertion that the women willingly acquiesced – or directly insisted upon – preservation after death, there is a strong implication that their willingness to be exhibited in life might be translated into a desire to continue that exhibition after death.

Elsewhere in accounts of female mummies, we find suggestions that, while the woman may not have directly expressed a wish to be embalmed/mummified/taxidermied, the 'art of embalming' offered a service that, perhaps, was to her benefit. George Head's description of the Egyptian damsel and the Mancunian old maid refers to the 'services of the toilet' that had erased signs of age in the two corpses – 'to which ladies are said to be particular' – and the advert for the Peruvian mummy displayed in Rochester draws a strange connection between Captain Woods riding through the wilderness of Peru and the helpless young woman buried alive by the Incas. Both have faced 'the risk of falling sacrifice to the resentment of the natives', casting Captain Woods's removal of the body almost as a daring rescue of damsel-in-distress by a dashing explorer on horseback.

All this returns us, at last, to the body of Miss Beswick.

The body in the Peter Street museum seems to have been immune to the sexualization and eroticization that we see in the other cases discussed in this chapter. I would suggest that this is, in part, the result of the perceived age of the woman on death. One of the constants in accounts of Miss Beswick is that she was 'old'. Head calls her an 'old maid'; Kohl calls her '*Mrs* Beswick', which is perhaps an acknowledgement of her age, but it certainly serves to remove an idea of her as an object of potential sexual fascination.

However, the lack of erotic othering in the case of Miss Beswick may also be the result of the perceived class of the woman. Another significant constant in all accounts is that she was rich. Head calls her a 'lady'; Kohl claims she was wealthy enough to leave her doctor an annual income of £500; Ashton uses the word 'affluent' and says she left her doctor a property of 'considerable value'; de Quincey claims that she was rich enough to bequeath her doctor £25,000. Unlike Saartje Baartman, who died penniless, or Miss Johnson, who may have died of tuberculosis in a syphilis hospital, Miss Beswick was a member of the landed gentry or aristocracy (assumed from the repeated word 'lady') who may have been, in today's money, a multi-millionaire.

For all my attempts to 'read' Miss Beswick alongside other contemporaneous female corpses, one of these things is not like the others. Unlike the other embalmed women discussed here, Miss Beswick was never presented as 'inferior' to the viewer. In fact, by the repeated emphasis on her wealth and class, viewers of her body were reminded that she was actually their social superior.

This is underlined further by the consistent efforts of writers to distance Miss Beswick from any man who might claim ownership of her body. Throughout the cases of Asroni, the Peruvian mummies in both Manchester and Rochester, Maria van Butchell, Miss Johnson, Saartje Baartman and Julia Pastrana, the idea of male ownership of the female body (in life and in death) looms large. Miss Johnson's dead body was the property of John Sheldon, with the descriptor in the Hunterian Museum stating this as fact until its destruction in 1941. Asroni's body was acquired, stripped of its cerements and donated by the Garnetts, just as the Peruvian mummy in Manchester was donated by Mr Stubbs. Captain Woods rode off with the Rochester body on the back of his horse, and Julia Pastrana's body was sold, bought and sold again by Theodore Lent.

In life, Maria van Butchell would have had no legal existence of her own, as the doctrine of coverture in English common law meant that her legal rights were subsumed by those of her husband on marriage, and she would have been unable to own property in her own right. Julia

Pastrana was married to Theodore Lent in the United States, which also observed the doctrine of coverture, though it was beginning to be dismantled during Pastrana's lifetime. In 1869, Harriet Beecher Stowe described the situation of married women in the United States thus:

> [T]he position of a married woman ... is, in many respects, precisely similar to that of the negro slave. She can make no contract and hold no property; whatever she inherits or earns becomes at that moment the property of her husband ... Though he acquired a fortune through her, or though she earn a fortune through her talents, he is the sole master of it, and she cannot draw a penny [...] [I]n the English common law a married woman is nothing at all. She passes out of legal existence.[17]

If Miss Johnson did indeed die at the Lock Hospital, then her status on death was as an inmate rather than a patient. The Lock wasn't so much a medical facility as an institution to house 'penitent Magdalenes afflicted with disease [syphilis], or sincerely desirous of abandoning the "primrose path that leads to the everlasting bonfire"'.[18]

Miss Beswick – in all accounts – is resolutely unmarried. She is a 'testatrix', meaning she has complete control over the disposal of her property, including (allegedly) her mortal remains. She is no inmate of a penitential institution, but rather someone with the agency and financial independence to employ a 'medical advisor' who, it transpires, was 'the most eminent surgeon by much in the North of England'. However, even that man is erased from the story, being relegated simply to the status of the man who embalmed the mummy in exchange for some cold, hard cash. While Kohl's account suggests that Dr White 'owned' the body of Miss Beswick – he was legally allowed to 'bequeath' it to the museum – this situation was simply the necessary circumstance through which Miss Beswick could 'take her place' alongside the antiquities of Egypt and Peru.

Imagine being a member of the Mechanics' Institute in 1840s Manchester and paying your sixpence (or threepence) to enter the museum on a day off from work, only to be confronted by the spectre of a woman who, like you, lived in Manchester. But while you've worked hard to earn your sixpence entrance fee, she had enough money to give her doctor £25,000 for the sake of an eccentric whim and enough property to leave a will disposing of it. The only superiority you could hope to feel under those circumstances would come from the fact that you are alive and she is dead.

* * *

For all the waxing lyrical of travel writers and advertising copywriters, it is important to remember that the exhibits under discussion in this chapter were all human corpses, embalmed, stuffed, dried and treated. The word 'mummy' is used somewhat euphemistically in the poetic descriptions of these bodies to obscure the reality of what is on display: a corpse.

The grotesque nature of such a display did not go unremarked by all visitors to the nineteenth-century museum. In 1834, Thomas Joseph Pettigrew included a chapter on 'Modern Embalmings' in his *History of Egyptian Mummies*, offering a summary of the methods of William Hunter, who was allegedly responsible for the preservation of Maria van Butchell (though his brother John is also sometimes credited with the work). Pettigrew's description of Maria van Butchell, who is reduced to 'the wife of a well-known eccentric character', states that it was 'properly speaking, a dessicated, rather than an embalmed body'.[19]

A visitor to the Hunterian Museum in 1857 offered an even more haunting assessment of the displayed corpse:

> No doubt extraordinary pains were taken to preserve both form and feature; and yet, what a wretched mockery of a once lovely woman it now appears, with its shrunken and rotten-looking bust, its hideous, mahogany coloured face, and its remarkably fine set of teeth. Between the feet are the remains of a green parrot – whether immolated or not at the death of his mistress is uncertain; but as it still retains its plumage, it is a far less repulsive object than the larger biped.[20]

This description lacks the claims of lifelikeness seen in other commentaries, with a suggestion that this is a 'mockery' of the human form. The slyly humorous nature of the reference to the 'remarkably fine set of teeth' (van Butchell's husband was a dentist, and her body had previously been displayed in his waiting room) and the arch parenthetical statement on the parrot, strips the displayed corpse of any semblance of dignity. By 1885, the body was described in the *Dictionary of*

National Biography as 'a repulsive-looking object', removing any final shred of humanity that may have clung to it.[21]

The dehumanization of the exhibited body is even more apparent in the case of women who weren't fully considered human in life, let alone in death. Charles Darwin wrote about the case of Julia Pastrana in his work, *The Variation of Animals and Plants Under Domestication*, stating:

> Julia Pastrana, a Spanish dancer, was a remarkably fine woman, but she had a thick masculine beard and a hairy forehead; she was photographed, and her stuffed skin was exhibited as a show; but what concerns us is, that she had in both the upper and lower jaw an irregular double set of teeth, one row being placed within the other, of which Dr Purland took a cast. From the redundancy of the teeth her mouth projected, and her face had a gorilla-like appearance.[22]

The reference to the 'gorilla-like appearance' and the subject matter of the book in which this statement appears might remind us that the body of Saartje Baartman was preserved by a zookeeper, not a surgeon, and that both women were objects of scientific scrutiny by those who believed they belonged to a different species.

It is clear that the experience of viewing the preserved corpse differed between visitors, which might encourage us to take the more poetic musings on dead female bodies with something of a pinch of salt. The advertisements for the Peruvian mummy in Rochester and the exhibition of Julia Pastrana's body in Piccadilly both include an assertion that there is nothing 'unpleasant' or 'indecent' about the exhibition – a statement so categoric one wonders what criticism they are pre-empting.

In the descriptions of bodies on display in Manchester's Peter Street museum there is little sense of the grotesquerie behind the cases, and we have no record of how the average museum visitor experienced the bodies on display. However, it's possible to perceive a tendency to dehumanization in the disregard shown towards the Peruvian mummy. Ashton's *Visits* simply notes that it was 'merely dipped in bitumen and buried in a sack of sand', a far cry from the romantic marketing of Captain Woods and his 'perfect' damsel.[23] And, anachronism aside, we may consider our own experience of viewing preserved human remains in museums: do we experience a romantic tendency to view mummies for their lifelike perfection? Or is our initial reaction one of horror and distaste at the ancient corpse with which we are confronted?

As I've said, Miss Beswick is treated somewhat differently to her sisters in post-mortem preservation, with descriptions of her body continuously evoking domesticity and intimacy rather than othering and exoticization. She is always a 'lady *of Manchester*' – preserved by the 'services of the toilet' at her own eccentric behest. There's no suggestion that she isn't human (in life or in death), or that she was preserved as an object of scientific research, reinforced by the subtle erasure of the 'most eminent surgeon by much in the North of England' from the narrative of her preservation. Unlike with Miss Johnson, there's no hint that Miss Beswick was the subject of dissection for medical research, or that Mr White – a man who 'measured innumerable skulls amongst the omnigenous seafaring population of Liverpool' – might have done anything other than politely attend to his patient's final wishes.

And yet, we might read a subtle undermining of the woman's status in some of the visitor accounts of viewing her corpse. The constant return to Miss Beswick as 'eccentric testatrix' leaves a question mark over the woman's state of mind, and a question mark that will prove very difficult to erase over the subsequent centuries. There's also something of a gap, as all the accounts gloss over the period between her request to be embalmed and the display of her corpse in a museum open to the general public.

There is a small but telling detail in George Head's account of viewing the body in the King Street museum. Although his description focuses on the pseudo-domestic vision of Asroni and Miss Beswick sitting together as an inter-generational pair linked by their femininity as much as by their existence as unburied cadavers, Head does give some small physical details about the appearance of Miss Beswick's body: she was 'not in fashionable costume, but enveloped from head to foot, in a dress of blue striped ticking, [...] fitting her so tightly, that it is probable the doctor first paid her over from top to toe with hot glue, and then drew on the garment'.[24]

The covering of hot glue transforms the display, momentarily, from a human body into an object (with the material value of £50, according to the Natural History Society's valuations), just as we saw with the description of Maria van Butchell's body. But it's the 'dress of blue striped ticking' that really captures the attention. Ticking is a tightly woven upholstery fabric, most commonly used for covering mattresses as its close weave prevents stuffing escaping through the fabric. For a 'lady of Manchester', more accustomed, perhaps, to Brussels lace, a tabby gown or a grey silk negligée, to be wrapped head-to-foot in a mattress cover and put on show for the town might be considered somewhat degrading.

In his assessment of the case of Miss Beswick in 1913, Francis Nicholson, following the (by then) established narrative of the woman's taphophobia, concluded: 'If Miss Beswick had known that her corpse would be gazed at by Manchester crowds in a Natural History Museum she would, I fancy, have preferred the risk of being buried alive to the ungenteel fate of being a specimen in a museum.'[25]

4

What was her name?

At the 1864 annual general meeting (AGM) of the Manchester Natural History Society, concerns were raised about the future of the Peter Street museum. In some ways, the museum had become a victim of its own success, with acquisitions over the three decades of its existence outstripping the capacity of its premises. The report of the meeting states: '[T]he collections are already so large as to be inconveniently crowded in the building; that the modes in which they are now conserved and exhibited are very imperfect and unsatisfactory.'[1]

One of the reasons for this overcrowding was that, in 1851, the Natural History Society had entered into what has been called an 'uneasy alliance' with the Manchester Geological Society, seeing the latter society's collections transported to the Peter Street museum from their former home at the residence of James Heywood on Mosley Street. This required the construction of additional rooms at the Peter Street museum, and it led to rows over 'access to specimens, admission to the museum, and even charges for custody of umbrellas'.[2]

Nevertheless, the overcrowding and somewhat fractious relationship with the Geological Society appears to have been managed reasonably well until the mid-1860s. Reports of the society periodically mention a problem with moths (kept under control by the curatorial staff), and the increased visitor numbers required the employment of additional staff, such as Mrs Reynolds, who was employed as 'door-keeper and general attendant on visitors' in 1857.[3]

Accounts of the state of the museum in the 1860s, written after the fact, tend to focus on the general dilapidation of its displays. Francis

Nicholson, for instance, states that: 'The neglect, due primarily to the impecuniosity of the Society in its later years, had resulted in many of the specimens of birds and mammals becoming moth-eaten and of insects becoming faded. A great number of the specimens had thus to be discarded.'[4] These accounts, however, are written with hindsight. In 1864, the Natural History Society laid the blame for the museum's struggles at a different door. The AGM report states bleakly that: '[O]f late the competition, so to speak, of the large and handsome *Free* Museum of the Salford Corporation at Peel Park has greatly diminished the public recourse to the Peter-Street Institution.'[5]

It's almost impossible to explain the relationship between Manchester and Salford to anyone who hasn't lived in either city. And both are now cities – Manchester was granted city status in 1853, and Salford in 1926 – though they neighbour each other so closely as to occasionally be fused into one in people's minds. Manchester was originally a township in the Salford Hundred, a subdivision of the historic county of Lancashire that retained its own court until the nineteenth century. Salford is now a borough of Greater Manchester, a metropolitan county formed in 1974 under the provisions of the Local Government Act 1972. Manchester and Salford retain their own elected city councils – Manchester's dating back to 1838, and Salford's to 1844 – and there are subtle differences in their respective administration of local government. However, there's almost no discernible difference or hard border between the two territories, and it's easy to pass between the two (or, indeed, stand in one or the other) without any awareness that you have moved to an entirely different city. Manchester has a reputation for 'appropriating' Salford's cultural assets – for example, iconic Mancunian Tony Wilson, founder of Factory Records, actually grew up in Salford. On the other hand, iconic Salfordian L. S. Lowry actually grew up in Manchester. So the relationship has some reciprocity and is, in the words of historian Nikolaus Pevsner, 'one of the most curious anomalies of England'.[6]

In 1864, Salford and Manchester existed much as they do now, two towns with city ambitions, sharing a territory and a history but operating independently of one another in terms of local government and municipal decisions. For the purposes of our story, a significant difference lies in their respective response to the Museums Act of 1845.

This piece of legislation empowered the town councils of larger municipal boroughs (those with a population of 10,000 or more) to raise funds via taxation for the foundation of free libraries and museums to serve their populace. Salford's town council took advantage of this legislation; Manchester's town council did not, though it clearly considered the idea, as reports of a potential municipal museum were published as early as August 1845.[7]

Salford Council had acquired the house and gardens at Lark Hill, an estate built by Colonel James Ackers in 1809 and subsequently owned by William Garnett (one of the brothers who donated the Egyptian mummy known as Asroni to the Natural History Society), in 1844. Garnett sold the Lark Hill estate to Manchester and Salford's (joint) Committee for Public Walks, Gardens and Playgrounds for £5,000, and it was converted into a public park, named Peel Park, in recognition of financial contributions from Robert Peel, the former prime minister and founder of the modern Conservative Party. In 1849, Salford Council raised money (through taxation and subscriptions) to transform the house into a public museum and library, and the building was opened as the Royal Museum and Public Library in 1850.

In the first year of its existence, the Royal Museum and Public Library (also known as the Peel Park Museum) welcomed visitors with extensive refreshment rooms and a library of over 12,000 volumes, many of which were available to be borrowed for free, making this the first free public lending library in the country. The building was extended in 1852 to include a large reading room, additional museum galleries and a new staircase to better accommodate visitors. And by 1864, Manchester's museum admitted it was struggling to compete.

One of the differences between the two museums was that Salford's museum was free to visit, while Manchester's was not. You may remember that the Natural History Society committee had considered the impact of its entrance fee in 1863, reflecting on the fact that, when the museum was opened for free in celebration of the Prince of Wales's marriage, 'more than six thousand people passed through the building'. The success of the Peel Park Museum, less than a mile and a half away, proves that it was right to think about 'what would be the popularity of the Museum if it could be thrown open to the general public free'.[8]

The problem for the Natural History Society was that, while Salford Corporation could operate a museum without an entrance fee, it didn't have sufficient funds to do so. The society's other source of income – subscriptions from members – had been declining for some time, as membership numbers gradually decreased.[9] It couldn't afford to lose the income from visitor fees as well.

At some point after the 1864 AGM, the Natural History Society realized the obvious solution to its problem. While Salford Corporation had taken advantage of the provisions of the Museums Act, Manchester Corporation was yet to do so. It decided to offer its collections to the Corporation as the foundation of a new free museum for the people of Manchester.

The society considered its offer to be a 'noble gift' to the city, and yet, to its consternation, Manchester Corporation turned it down. The response to this rejection detailed in the report of the 1866 AGM makes it clear what the society's vision of a free museum for Manchester was:

> Had the Corporation accepted the noble gift which the Society was prepared to make over, and with it the continuous assistance in the management of the Museum of gentlemen who would have been carefully selected from amongst the most cultivated and competent men of the district, there is little doubt but that in a short time Manchester would have been distinguished by the possession, and honoured for supporting, a splendid *free museum on a recognized scientific basis*, on a scale as yet unknown out of the metropolis. Such an institution placed, perhaps, in a public park, could not fail to have afforded to the intelligent population of this neighbourhood, educational opportunities and influences of very great value, especially among the daily increasing class of thoughtful persons, who seek for their recreation a more systematic cultivation than can be afforded by the over-crowded and imperfectly arranged curiosities of an ordinary Free Museum.[10]

Hubris aside, this statement – as well as the surviving correspondence between the society and Manchester Corporation – reveals the source of the disagreement between the two parties. While the Natural History Society was planning to make a 'noble gift' of its collection to the local municipal body, it was with the condition that it would give 'continuous assistance in the management of the Museum' and select the curatorial team. Manchester Corporation was willing to accept the former, but not the latter, insisting that it would be in full control of the management of any future museum for the city, including the selection of staff.

It was an impasse that was never overcome, with the Natural History Society growing increasingly frustrated by the Corporation's refusal to accept that a museum should be arranged, primarily, on a 'recognized scientific basis', and the Corporation refusing to budge on its insistence on controlling the curation of the hypothetical museum itself.

As can be seen from the statement in 1866, the Natural History Society suggested that the Corporation may want to follow Salford's example and house the new municipal museum in a public park. The two locations suggested were Philips Park and Queen's Park, which had been opened in 1846 on the same day as Peel Park in Salford. In negotiations with the Corporation, the Natural History Society drew attention to the success of the Peel Park Museum, arguing that Manchester could create something even better than Salford in Queen's Park (to the north of the town centre) or Philips Park (to the east).[11]

When the negotiations with Manchester failed, the society came up with a Plan B. If Manchester didn't want the collection, then perhaps Salford would. Salford Corporation already had a museum, and so the 'noble gift' of the society's collection could augment the existing museum. Peel Park was physically closer to Peter Street than Queen's Park or Philips Park, and so the move would potentially make more sense.

It appears that Plan B was never pursued in earnest by the Natural History Society, and no correspondence between the society and the Salford Corporation survives, so it isn't clear whether the 'noble gift' was ever formally offered to Salford. There are hints in later reports that the society realized that it would encounter the same opposition from Salford as it had from Manchester, particularly in relation to the management and curation of the collection. There also seems to have been concern about the size of the Natural History Society's collection (which had already outgrown its purpose-built museum on Peter Street) and the difficulty of transferring that to a museum that already had a substantial collection of its own. An appendix to the report of the 1866 Natural History Society AGM notes that only a 'certain portion of the objects now exhibited by the society' would have been suitable for 'display in some Free Museum'.[12]

By 1865, the Manchester Natural History Society had a large collection of natural history specimens, antiquities and curiosities, as well as a building and staff to maintain, and its income simply couldn't meet the expense. If a municipal home could not be found for the collections, then perhaps an academic home could be found instead.

* * *

Manchester Grammar School, founded in 1515 by Hugh Oldham with the assistance of Hugh Bexwycke and his mother Joan, continued to be the pre-eminent seat of learning for the upper middle classes of Manchester throughout the nineteenth century.[13] This was the school to which Thomas de Quincey was sent at the beginning of the century, though the teaching at that point was 'dated' and lacked the scientific curriculum that was required by 'the new and large industrial class, along with the merchant class' (i.e. the class of men who founded Manchester's intellectual associations and societies). The governors of the school at the time – the 'Feoffes' – were largely members of the landed gentry who viewed the school as something of a finishing school for young gentlemen.[14] In 1849, the Manchester Grammar School was merged with the town's commercial school (founded in the 1830s) and the Feoffes all resigned, creating an institution called the Manchester Free Grammar School that was intended to provide a modern scientific education for the wealthy middle classes, as well as subsidized places (bursaries) for the less wealthy. The school would now educate boys up to the age of fourteen who were intended for 'commercial careers', and boys up to the age of nineteen who were intended for university.

The problem, in the 1840s, was that boys educated at the Manchester Grammar School had to leave the town in order to attend university. This had been a bone of contention for some time prior to 1849, as the school had long admitted boarders from outside Manchester – or, indeed, outside Lancashire – who would get an 'endowment' from the school and head off to Oxbridge on Manchester money.[15] But of course, even local students had to head off to Oxbridge after completing their studies – or, perhaps, to Scotland – as there wasn't anywhere else for them to go.

By the time of the industrial revolution, the UK only had six universities (meaning institutions incorporated under royal charter and given the power to award degrees): the Universities of Oxford and Cambridge in England, and the Universities of St Andrews, Glasgow, Aberdeen and Edinburgh in Scotland. In 1826, the London University was founded, and this institution was incorporated by royal charter as University College, London in 1836, by which time another institution, King's College, London (founded in 1829), had also received its royal charter. The two colleges became the first constituent colleges of the University of London, the first 'modern' English university, with the power to confer degree in arts, law and medicine but not theology, which remained the province of Oxford, Cambridge and, from 1832, Durham.[16]

What Manchester lacked in the first half of the nineteenth century – as was the case with all the urbanized, industrialized areas outside London – was an establishment focused on what we now call higher education. Various institutions – including the Lit and Phil, the Royal Manchester Institution (established in 1823 and focused on the exhibition of fine art, though its building on Mosley Street also housed a laboratory under the management of Professor of Chemistry Lyon Playfair), the Manchester Mechanics' Institute and its counterpart in Salford (established in 1839) and the Phrenological Society and its associated museum, Mr Bally's Gallery of Casts – offered teaching in the form of both public lectures and classes for scholars. There were also a number of libraries in the town with collections that could supplement an academic programme, though the Portico and the Atheneum were only open to members, Chetham's Library, while open to the public, was 'not so well known, or at least made so extensively available, as it ought to be', and the public circulating libraries in Manchester and Salford were focused on popular, rather than academic, material.[17] None of these institutions and organizations could do what the University of London could do: teach and award degrees in its own right.

The earliest attempt to address this gap in Manchester occurred in 1783, pre-dating the foundation of the London universities by decades. Members of the Lit and Phil, which had been established two years earlier, proposed the establishment of the College of Arts and Sciences in Manchester:

> This INSTITUTION is intended to provide a Course of LIBERAL INSTRUCTION, compatible with the Engagements of COMMERCIAL LIFE, favourable to all its higher Interests, and at the same Time, preparatory to the Systematic Studies of the UNIVERSITY. To unite *Philosophy* with *Art*, the moral and intellectual culture of the *mind*, with the pursuits of *fortune*, and to superadd the noblest powers of *enjoyment*, to the *acquisition* of *wealth*, are the GREAT OBJECTS, which it professes to hold in view. THESE OBJECTS bear no relation to PARTIES, either in RELIGION or POLITICS.[18]

Lectures were to be given on mathematics by Henry Clarke, chemistry by Thomas Henry, and arts, ethics and law by Rev. Thomas Barnes, and these would be arranged into a 'session' (a course) delivered from October 1783 to April 1794. The college would run four of these sessions, at a charge of two guineas each or six guineas for all four.

In September 1783, the College of Arts and Sciences was able to advertise an already expanded programme. Henry Clarke was out, replaced by James Dinwiddie, but there was now a course on fine arts by George Bew and Dinwiddie's lectures on geography, chronology and natural history would also be offered to ladies 'at a separate hour'. The president of the college in September 1783 was Thomas Percival, one of the founders of the Lit and Phil, and the governors included George Bew, James Dinwiddie, Thomas Henry and Charles White.[19] The latter, who had already gained a reputation as 'the most eminent surgeon by much in the North of England', gave lectures on anatomy for the college in October 1786: 'Further Particulars and printed Proposals for delivering these Courses, may be had gratis, at Mr *White*'s, and Mr *Henry*'s Houses in King-street, or at Dr *White*'s Anatomical Museum, in Cross-street.'[20]

To the modern eye, the College of Arts and Sciences can seem like an institution way ahead of its time, and it has been described as the 'first institution of its kind in the country'.[21] But it seems that the country wasn't ready for it, as the college only lasted five years before being dissolved and its courses ended, due, according to one commentator, to 'a superstitious dread of the tendency of science to unfit young men for the ordinary details of business'.[22] In his consideration of the college, William Charles Henry (grandson of its founder Thomas Henry) suggests that the institution was never intended to be an academic one, or anything approaching a university, but rather a series of evening classes 'to occupy, in a rational and instructive manner, the evening leisure of young men, whose time, during the day, was devoted to commercial employments', like a sort of white-collar Mechanics' Institute.[23] This is undermined somewhat by the college's own advertisements, in which the scale and ambition of the project is made clear: its courses, while not higher education in themselves, would serve as appropriate 'preparatory' study for university, while at the same time being 'compatible' with commercial life.

The ambition stated by the founders of the College of Arts and Sciences is not dissimilar to the argument made for the foundation of the University of London, albeit some forty years ahead of it. In 1825, poet Thomas Campbell wrote:

> Wealth, whether small or great, should always be connected with instruction, and the great means of attaining this end is to have proper institutions of education [...] It may be that all the means of education are, by some means or other, to be got at in London: but a man would wear out his shoes in trudging about to explore them [...] let it suffice to say, that no academy can answer the purposes of a well founded university.[24]

The problem that Campbell explores in this proposal for a new university in London is the exact same one that the men of Manchester were trying to solve in 1783. The huge expansion of the middle class (or merchant class or industrial class), who were now often far wealthier than members of the landed gentry, meant that the education system needed to adapt to better serve their needs.

While London got its university in 1836, the failure of Manchester's College of Arts and Sciences left a gap in the second city that wouldn't be filled for several decades.

* * *

Manchester had another go at creating a secular university college that would meet the needs of the merchant and manufacturing classes in 1851.

John Owens was a Manchester businessman, the son of Owen Owens of Flintshire, who was a manufacturer of hat linings, and a 'currier and furrier'.[25] The life of John Owens appears to have been fairly unremarkable, and very few details are known. His will, however, was a game-changer.

When he died in 1846, Owens left a sizeable bequest, including a series of conditions and instructions, for the endowment of a new college in Manchester. The outline of what the new college should be like has been described as 'a plain Manchester merchant's ideal of what he would like a college in a great town to be'.[26] Reflecting on the first hundred years of the college's existence, Henry Buckley Charlton summarized this 'ideal' in this way:

> The college is to be a non-residential institution primarily for teaching. Its teaching is to include branches of knowledge as are, or may be, recognised university subjects; it is teaching meant specifically for the people of its own region and mainly, therefore, for a new social group. For many, if not most, of these it would be the only means of systematic higher education: the older universities were too far away and otherwise too expensive; moreover, Oxford and Cambridge were only open to them, even if they had means to go there, if their conscience allowed them to subscribe to the Anglican creed. Finally, Owens was to be a college for the education of males.[27]

This description of the ideal 'college in a great town' bears some comparison with the ambitions of the College of Arts and Sciences in the 1780s, as well as the principles that underpinned the foundation of the London University in 1826. The reference to the 'Anglican creed' is also a reminder that a large number of the men involved in the development of Manchester's academic and political scene – including key members of the Lit and Phil, the Portico Library, Manchester Town Council and the Mechanics' Institute – were non-conformists, Unitarians and Wesleyans, some of whom (like Thomas Henry Robinson, the man who bought John Leigh Philips's cabinet of insects) had been involved in the foundation of another Manchester academic institution, the Manchester Academy, a theological college for 'Dissenters' that also included a scientific and literary curriculum.[28]

The trustees of John Owens's will set to work realizing his vision, and a college was opened in 1851, operating out of a building on Quay

Street that had formerly been the residence of Richard Cobden. In its first year, the college had sixty-two students on its books.[29] The following year, it started to admit part-time students, and in 1859 it had fifty-seven day students and seventy-seven part-time students, and the college was approved as a provincial examination centre for matriculation candidates for the University of London.

In its early years, the majority of the college's intake were part-time students, attending evening sessions outside of employment or preparation for employment. The college admitted students from around the age of fourteen, and it seems the average age was on the lower end for the first few years, until the degree regulation from the University of London raised the age of matriculation from fourteen to sixteen. Colin Lees and Alex Robertson have suggested that this focus on part-time, evening sessions meant that the new college 'differed little from the Mechanics' Institute'.[30] I would add that it also differed little from the earlier College of Arts and Sciences in this respect, and there is some evidence that Owens College encountered the same 'superstitious dread of the tendency of science to unfit young men for the ordinary details of business'. One account of a 'typical' interview with the parents of prospective students paraphrased a father's demands: 'I am a calico printer, or a dyer, or a brewer, and I want you to teach my son chemistry so far, and so far only, as it is at once applicable to my trade.'[31]

This state of affairs continued for pretty much the first twenty years of the college's existence. Owens College, however, like so many of the Manchester institutions we've encountered so far, had ambitions.

In many ways, Owens College had to come up with its own plan to realize those ambitions. As Lees and Robertson have pointed out, there were no examples that the college could follow: 'Of the four English universities Oxford and Cambridge were ancient collegiate foundations, King's College and University College, London, were metropolitan and Durham was recent, small and predominantly theological.'[32] It's generally acknowledged that Owens College was more influenced in its foundation and subsequent operation by the Scottish universities, particularly Glasgow, which had been established earlier but with an approach more suited to the needs of an industrial town.

By the 1860s, the trustees of Owens College were looking to expand. An Owens College Expansion Committee was set up, who actively raised funds to develop the college, citing overcrowded classrooms and the need to expand their student base from beyond the immediate environs of the college to the wider 'region of Manchester'. It was probably obvious from the start that the Quay Street premises would never properly suffice for the college, as in its second year of operation (1852), the college's prizegiving ceremonies had to be held at the Town Hall on King Street and the Royal Manchester Institution on Mosley Street.[33] Owens College was always going to need a bigger building.

The Expansion Committee worked out what to do in 1867. If sufficient funds could be raised, a new building could be erected for the college. They set their sights on land in Chorlton-on-Medlock, a former township to the south of Manchester, which had been incorporated into the new borough of Manchester in 1838. John Owens himself had lived at Nelson Street, a well-to-do street to the south of the township, just off the turnpike road to Oxford. Chorlton-on-Medlock had seen a lot of development, beginning in 1793–94 when the formerly rural area was divided up on a grid system and sold to wealthy landowners, and continuing through the early nineteenth century which saw the erection of cotton mills at the northern edge of the township (along with the associated poor quality workers' housing, particularly in the area known as Little Ireland) and the establishment of large houses for millowners and merchants at its southern edge, such as those on Nelson Street. Despite this, there was still land up for grabs, and at a lower price than in the town centre. In December 1867, the Expansion Committee had identified a potential plot in Chorlton-on-Medlock, which lay in between Burlington Street and Coupland Street, and a member of the committee, Thomas Ashton (*not* the Thomas Ashton who wrote about the Peter Street museum, but rather a wealthy industrialist who served as a leading figure in the college's expansion), bought the land in trust for Owens College. The following year, the Committee would appoint architect Alfred Waterhouse to design the new premises for Owens College, and the foundation stone would be laid by the Duke of Devonshire in September 1870.

And this was all very fortuitous timing, because just as Owens College was laying down the payment for the Chorlton-on-Medlock site, a certain Natural History Society was on the hunt for a new home for its collection.

* * *

By the time the Manchester Natural History Society had exhausted its attempts to find a municipal home for its museum, the potential for an academic home was (for the first time ever) a very real possibility. The society offered its 'noble gift' to Owens College and entered into negotiations that were substantially shorter than the back-and-forth with Manchester Corporation. Perhaps it was desperation, or perhaps the society was more convinced that the college would be amenable to arranging a new museum on a 'scientific basis', but the society conceded to a compromise position fairly quickly. The collection would be transferred to Owens College, which would oversee the management of a new museum; however, the college agreed to the society's condition that the museum would be open to the public, and not just to students at the college.

In 1868, the Manchester Natural History Society began the process of dissolving the society and transferring its collection to Owens College. It appointed a board of 'Commissioners', led by Robert Dukinfield Darbishire, to manage the collection and supervise the disposal of the society's property and, with that, the Natural History Society came to an end.

If all of this sounds rather simple, it really wasn't. The Peter Street museum was a large building, packed with display cabinets containing everything from a Burmese Idol to the skull of a sixty-two-year-old workhorse. The building itself had to be sold, and the vast array of exhibits and artefacts had to be prepared for removal to a building that didn't yet exist. The first meeting of the Commissioners took place in March 1868, less than three months after Owens College had purchased the land in Chorlton-on-Medlock and nine months before it would appoint an architect. The Peter Street museum would stay open for the first couple of years of the transition, under the curation of Thomas Alcock, who had taken over after the death of Captain Brown in 1862, and a new doorkeeper, Sarah Burkes, was appointed in 1869, suggesting that the museum was still open to visitors.[34]

In the background, though, the Commissioners were working out what to do about the exhibits, which, as Johan Georg Kohl had pointed out back in 1844, were a 'barbarous' mixture of natural history, antiquity, ethnography, archaeology and, of course, curiosity.

The agreement with Owens College covered the natural history specimens, aside from those which, as Francis Nicholson noted, were so 'moth-eaten' or 'faded' that they had to be destroyed. The Commissioners also noted that many of the mammal specimens were 'old and very dirty' and that 'some are atrociously stuffed', before recommending the destruction or removal of many of them.[35] On the other hand, the insect specimens – the cabinet of insects that had formed the foundation of the Natural History Society's earliest museum – were mostly transferred over to the college's ownership, with the exception of those that were too faded to rescue.

In terms of the antiquities and curiosities, it's hard to discern the exact reasons for the decisions taken by the Commissioners in their records, and so conjecture has to be made. The Peruvian Mummy was not transferred to Owens College, but the body of Asroni and the associated sarcophagi were. I have to assume that this decision was taken due to the perceived value – both in cultural and monetary terms – of the respective exhibits. Slightly more puzzling is the decision taken about the horses on display in the Peter Street museum. The skull of sexagenarian equine Old Billy *was* transferred to the college, but the stuffed body of Napoleon's charger Vizier was not. The French horse was, after some discussion with the Foreign Office, offered to the 'Emperor of the French', i.e. Napoleon III.[36] It really isn't clear what happened next, as a note that has survived on Vizier, written after the fact, states: 'From these extracts it appears evident that the packing-case containing the horse was dispatched to the Louvre in 1868 [...] but there is no record in the minutes of this, or of any acknowledgement from the Director of Imperial Museums.'[37]

Vizier – now known as Vizir – eventually made his way to the Musée de l'Armée in Paris (where he remains on display), after being stored and forgotten for nearly thirty years at the Louvre.[38] It remains unclear whether Napoleon III responded to the Commissioners in 1868. It's also not clear whether the Louvre was expecting the packing-case that arrived at its door shortly afterwards, given that it made no attempt to either display the body of the horse or thank the Manchester Commissioners for their noble gift.

The remaining curiosities (or most of them) were sold at auction on 8 October 1868:

> The collection of curiosities which Messrs. Capes and Dunn undertook to dispose of yesterday was a very curious one indeed. Many of the articles were brought to the hammer in such an alarming state of delapidation [*sic*], as to evoke expressions of derision from the tribe of brokers, to whom it is not given to see such a collection of what they term 'job lots' every day. Even the followers of Dr Dryasdust, and they were few in number, found it difficult to get up the faintest enthusiasm in the face of such shabby specimens. The auctioneers' porter, a man of impassable countenance, walked gravely about with one of the first lots, a dried human head, tattooed from New Zealand. The ghastly relic was in a tolerable state of preservation, but the demand for heads was slow, and it fetched only 18*s*. [...] Mr J. Plant, curator of the Peel Park museum, secured for that institution the large Burmese idol which stood in the entrance hall [...] A Peruvian mummy was next introduced. This repulsive object was no 'statue of flesh', as Horace Smith described the Egyptian mummy in Belzoni's collection, but a ghastly huddled heap of bones and dried flesh, from which the spectators turned with instinctive loathing. It was said to be many thousands of years old. Nineteen shillings was the value which was put upon it, and no higher bid could be obtained.[39]

All this brings us inexorably back to Miss Beswick, whose body was not one of the lots sold at the October auction, nor was it transferred to another museum. The Commissioners had a very different plan in mind for her.

* * *

Robert Dukinfield Darbishire (1826–1908) was a Mancunian lawyer and philanthropist. He was a Unitarian, like his father Samuel (who was one of the trustees of Cross Street Chapel, a founding member of both the Atheneum and the Manchester Academy, and a close friend of Elizabeth Gaskell's husband William), and had received his degree from the University of London in 1845. As a child, Robert

Dukinfield Darbishire played with Elizabeth Gaskell's children at their house on Plymouth Grove; in later life, he was one of the founders of the Whitworth Art Gallery and Manchester High School for Girls, being made a Freeman of the City of Manchester in 1899. But, when he was in his forties, Robert Dukinfield Darbishire was the first person to try and find out the true story of Miss Beswick, the Manchester Mummy.

He didn't have much information to go on. From the correspondence that survives, it appears that the only information Darbishire had about the body known as Miss Beswick were the short anecdotal accounts that I have related in previous chapters of this book. He certainly doesn't appear to have had any details of the provenance or acquisition by the Natural History Society – and he didn't even know the woman's identity.

What is abundantly clear from the records kept by the Commissioners and subsequently preserved in the Manchester Museum Archive, now part of the University of Manchester Special Collections, is that at no point did the Commissioners, led by Darbishire, consider the embalmed body of a Mancunian old maid to be an appropriate object for display in a museum. There is no question of this exhibit being transferred to Owens College, and no attempt to transfer or sell it to another museum or institution. The only option the Commissioners explored was the disposal of the artefact, but as it wasn't a badly stuffed monkey or a moth-eaten squirrel (though it may well have been both badly stuffed and moth-eaten at this stage), they don't appear to have considered simply destroying it.

I say 'it', but this suggests that Darbishire viewed the body of Miss Beswick as a material artefact to be dealt with like an antique coin or a fossil, and this wasn't the case at all. Darbishire's letters relating to Miss Beswick reveal that he viewed the body as just that, the body of a Mancunian woman that had remained unburied for some time after death. He didn't want to destroy Miss Beswick; he wanted to arrange her funeral.

The first indication of this approach comes in the notes of the first meeting of the Commissioners on 9 March 1868. Some preliminary work on the collections had already been carried out, including the first attempts to deal with the Miss Beswick problem. A note reads: 'Reported that no reply had been received to a communication to Mr Brown Clayton respecting the future custody of the body of Miss Beswick.'[40] Only one half of Darbishire's correspondence has survived – the letters written *by* him, not those written *to* him – so I have to surmise some of what follows. The 'communication to Mr Brown Clayton' has also not survived, so again I can only offer conjecture as to what it might have contained.

Mr Brown Clayton is, I deduce from the later correspondence, Richard Clayton Browne-Clayton, esq., of Adlington, Cheshire. Admittedly, this initially raises more questions than it answers, but Darbishire's thinking will soon become clear.

Richard Clayton Browne-Clayton was the son of Lieutenant General Robert Browne, who adopted the additional surname of Clayton after his marriage to Henrietta Clayton in 1803. Henrietta Clayton was the daughter of Sir Richard Clayton, baronet, and Ann White of Manchester. Ann White was the daughter of Dr Charles White, 'the most eminent surgeon by much in the North of England'. The Commissioners may not have known the identity of the Mancunian old maid, but they certainly knew the identity of the doctor who embalmed her.

On 1 April 1868, Darbishire wrote to a firm of solicitors, Messrs Shuttleworth and Sons, saying that he believed them to represent Mr Browne-Clayton and that he 'had had communications' from their client on the matter of Miss Beswick's body. In his letter, Darbishire describes Mr Browne-Clayton as the owner of property passed through 'the will of a late Miss Beswick' and that the preservation of Miss Beswick's body was 'a condition of the enjoyment of your client's predecessors [...] of some portion of the estate'.[41] On 29 June 1868, Darbishire wrote to a man named William Wilson stating:

> As I was informed that the coffin intended for Miss Beswick whose mummy is now in the Natural History Society Museum in Peter St is still in Mr Brown Clayton's stable, I shall be much obliged if you will inform me what was Miss Beswick's Christian name and in what year she died.[42]

Although we might guess that Darbishire wrote to Mr Browne-Clayton on the understanding that he was the great-grandson of Dr Charles

White, it's harder to work out where the story of the coffin in the stable came from.

There are two possibilities that I can suggest. The first is that an anecdotal story about Charles White inheriting property in Miss Beswick's will and keeping a coffin in the stable for her was circulating, but never published, during the display of her body in the Peter Street museum. It may be remembered that Thomas Ashton included the claim that Miss Beswick bequeathed 'a property of considerable value' to her medical advisor in his description of the museum exhibit. It is possible that he knew, but did not record, a story about an unused coffin in the stable.

The alternative is that Mr Browne-Clayton himself made the claims about the will and the coffin in the 'communications' Darbishire received from him prior to his letters to Messrs Shuttleworth and Sons.

Either way, no further information was forthcoming. In June 1868, Darbishire wrote to Messrs Shuttleworth and Son to request that their client take responsibility for the body of Miss Beswick. He also asked if they could provide him with the woman's name, the date of her will and the place where it was proved. On 25 June, the lawyers wrote back to him stating that their client had no knowledge of the date of Miss Beswick's will or where it was proved. They were also unable to furnish the Commissioners with the woman's Christian name, and they made no mention of the coffin in the stable.[43]

On 11 July, Darbishire wrote back to Messrs Shuttleworth and Son, thanking them for their letter and the lack of information and explaining that the Commissioners now intended to 'have the remains of the late Miss Beswick decently interred in one of the cemeteries near this town'. Presumably, Darbishire received no response from William Wilson, as he made one last attempt to learn the identity of the woman he was about to bury. In another letter dated 11 July, Darbishire wrote to a Miss Beswick and a Miss Boardman (no address details survive) saying that he understood 'she was a relation of yours' and asking, once again, for Miss Beswick's Christian name and the date of her death, as well as enquiring 'if there is any real objection to their having her remains decently buried'.[44]

I don't know which Miss Beswick or Miss Boardman Darbishire wrote to, but it certainly appears that they didn't answer him. No one was able to tell him the name of the Manchester Mummy.

However, as you may have noticed, Darbishire was no longer referring to the body as a 'mummy' in his letters, but rather as 'the remains of the late Miss Beswick'. She had ceased to be a museum exhibit to be disposed of, and had, instead, become the body of a dead woman to be 'decently interred'.

And this was the plan all along, of course. On 19 June, before his final attempts to learn some details about the woman, Darbishire had written to Thomas Alcock, curator of the Peter Street museum, stating that the 'Commissioners have decided to bury Miss Beswicke's remains' and that he had already asked Messrs Satterfield (a firm of undertakers) 'to make the necessary arrangements'.[45] His final letter to the enigmatic Miss Beswick and Miss Boardman was, it transpires, a last check that no family members would object to this unconventional funeral.

There were two further problems to overcome before the body of Miss Beswick could be laid to rest.

The first lay in the fact that you couldn't then – and can't now – bury a body in a cemetery without a certificate of death. In order to address this, Darbishire wrote to the Secretary of State for Home Affairs to request permission to conduct the unorthodox funeral. In his letter, Darbishire gave a brief overview of the story as he understood it:

> Many years ago – I have no particulars of the date – a Miss ___ Beswicke, for reasons which are not known now, desired that her body might be embalmed and kept above ground [...] Her body duly embalmed was, it is reported, long kept by her medical adviser, a Dr White, and was deposited into the hands of the Society, certainly upon the year 1833, and still remained with them until the beginning of the year it dissolved itself and handed its collection on to the Commissioners [...] The Commissioners do not wish to retain the remains and desire to bury them decorously.[46]

He then wrote to the Bishop of Manchester, including a slightly different version of the story:

> A certain Miss Beswicke who died many years ago, being afraid of being buried alive, or of being disinterred, arranged that her body should be embalmed and directed that it should be kept above ground.
>
> After several years – 30 or 40 – and about 30 years ago, by some arrangement or other, this dried up corpse was lodged in the Natural History Society's Museum in Peter St where it now is [...] The Commissioners wish to have these remains decently put away and propose to have them interred.[47]

It's very interesting that, in his letter to the Home Secretary, Darbishire reveals some knowledge of how the body ended up in the museum, but no knowledge of why the mummification happened. Yet, in his letter to the Bishop, he claims no knowledge of why the body was 'lodged' in the museum, but states firmly that Miss Beswick was 'afraid of being buried alive, or of being disinterred' (hedging his bets between taphophobia and body-snatching).

The Home Secretary wrote back to say that 'no certificate of death be necessary', and the Bishop of Manchester replied to say that Darbishire should simply arrange 'which ceremony he deems fitting', in response to a question as to whether there was a special form of service that should be observed under such unusual circumstances.

The Bishop's response leads us to the second problem that Darbishire had to overcome. As a Unitarian, he was unfamiliar with Anglican funeral services. On 19 June, he expressed his concern about this to another of the Commissioners, stating:

> I will arrange about Miss Beswicke, but I am not very familiar with the rites of the Church of England as to interments. If you think there is anything necessary beyond the usual appointment with the registrar and chaplain of the cemetery, please to drop me a line, at this office.[48]

In the end, Darbishire's concerns were all addressed and Messrs Satterfield were able to receive the body of Miss Beswick and prepare it for burial, though they were advised to 'please not go to any unnecessary expense in providing an oak coffin or otherwise', suggesting that the apocryphal coffin from Mr Browne-Clayton's stable never did make an appearance.

Darbishire arranged for the burial to take place in Manchester General Cemetery, a municipal cemetery in Harpurhey, North Manchester, on 22 July 1868. The name and date of death of the deceased were unknown, and no headstone was put up to mark the grave. The following month, the *Manchester Guardian* reported on the burial:

> A CURIOUS INTERMENT – 'On the 22d of July were committed to the earth in the Harpurhey Cemetery, the remains of Miss Beswick, removed from the Peter-street Museum.' There is a tradition that this lady, who is supposed to have died about 100 years ago, had acquired so strong a fear of being buried alive, that she left certain property to her medical

> attendant, so long, so the story runs, as she should be kept above ground. The doctor seems to have embalmed the body with tar, and then swathed it in a strong bandage, leaving the face exposed, and to have kept 'her' out of the grave as long as he could. For many years past the mummy had been lodged in the rooms of the Manchester Natural History Society, where it has long been an object of much popular interest. It seems that the Commissioners, who are charged with the re-arrangement of the Society's collections, have deemed this specimen undesirable, and have at last buried it.[49]

On 14 August 1868, Robert Dukinfield Darbishire, unable to find out who the woman actually was, submitted the invoice of Messrs Satterfield for 'Miss Beswick's funeral' to the treasurer of the Commission, and the anonymous old maid was 'at last' laid to rest.

But, as any fan of mummy stories is well aware, burial is only the beginning.

5

Madame Beswick's supernatural pranks

Miss Beswick had only been in her anonymous grave for five months when her story was resurrected with quite a different take on the tale.

Robert Dukinfield Darbishire had not been able to ascertain Miss Beswick's first name, but a man named James Dronsfield knew it. And what's more, he claimed not to be the only person who did.

In early January 1869, a pamphlet entitled *Ben Brierley's New Year's Gift* was advertised for sale, at tuppence an issue. Ben Brierley was a weaver-turned-journalist and Lancashire dialect writer who was born in Failsworth (in between Manchester and Oldham) in 1825. A self-taught writer, Brierley began to contribute articles about Lancashire life and 'character' to local papers in the 1850s, and in April 1869 he would launch his own regular publication, *Ben Brierley's Journal*, that would run monthly and then weekly until 1891. *Ben Brierley's New Year's Gift* was a precursor to the *Journal*, including a piece called 'Ab-o'th'-Yate's Christmas Dinner' – Ab-o'th'-Yate being a pseudonym or persona Brierley used in his writing, to conjure up the Lancastrian character.

Of interest for this story, though, is the fact that *Ben Brierley's New Year's Gift* also included a piece by James Dronsfield, which bore the title 'The Peter Street Mummy, a Legend of Birchen Bower'. In this story, which was republished by the *Oldham Chronicle* later in 1869, Dronsfield would not only name the mummy, but also reveal a very different reason for her post-mortem preservation.

The Peter Street Mummy was, in fact, Hannah Beswick, a wealthy woman from Hollinwood, near Oldham, who owned a house and estate called Birchen Bower. She was a well-known figure in the local area, known as Madame Beswick, but she was also eccentric. In 1745, when the army of Charles Edward Stuart (known as Bonnie Prince Charlie) was marching across the north of England in its attempted Jacobite invasion, Madame Beswick became terrified that they would steal her wealth and belongings, and so she hid them around Birchen Bower. After the Jacobite threat receded, Madame Beswick kept her treasure hidden, refusing to tell any of her family where her riches were.

On her death, she was embalmed by her family physician, Dr White, on her own instructions. Her brother had almost been buried alive after he fell into a trance, and as a result Madame Beswick feared a similar fate. However, the embalming served an additional purpose, as the doctor was instructed to return her preserved body to Birchen Bower every twenty-one years, so that she might inspect her hidden treasure from beyond the grave. Local legend stated that her body was taken to the granary and kept there for a week, during which time various supernatural occurrences might be witnessed. Eventually, the treasure was discovered by a weaver named 'Joe at Tamer's', who sold the gold in Manchester.

Dronsfield's story introduces a supernatural element that hadn't existed previously. While the Peter Street Mummy was 'curiosity', there is no record of any paranormal phenomena being associated with it. It was a material curiosity, rather than a ghost. I would suggest that it is the other element introduced in 'The Peter Street Mummy', a very specific – and very real – location that allows for the mummy to be transformed into a ghost. The poetically named Birchen Bower is a site that can be haunted, giving Madame Beswick a physical locus for post-mortem manifestation that is far more evocative than either the generic 'Manchester' (as in 'Manchester Mummy) or the modern and rational 'Peter Street museum'.

Madame Beswick was a mummy in the Peter Street museum, but she was a legend at Birchen Bower.

* * *

James Dronsfield was born in Hollinwood in 1826. He was a friend and collaborator of both Ben Brierley and Samuel Bamford, editing the work of the former, including collections of his Ab-o'th'-Yate stories. Dronsfield wrote his own sketches of Lancashire life, particularly drawing on the history of Oldham and Hollinwood, which he contributed to local papers under his own name and a penname, Jerry Lichenmoss. He also, like Brierley, published versions of local 'legends', such as 'Chamber Ho' Boggart', the story of an old hall on 'the southern slope of Oldham' that was haunted by a boggart, a troublesome spirit that caused mayhem for the hall's occupants.[1]

An important thing to note about Dronsfield's writing is that he never made any claim to invention or creation. Like Brierley and Bamford, Dronsfield cast his writing as collection and curation instead. In the 'Chamber Ho' Boggart' story, he is careful to describe the geography of the actual hall, assuming a level of familiarity on the part of his readers. He also both cites and names the local people who have supplied him with information. In the case of Chamber Hall, it is 'old Jenny Hathershaw' who is his main informant, 'a worthy dame, whose head was a storeroom, crammed full of ghosts, fairies and witches', but who was 'born on the estate' and 'her relatives have been tenants thereof for about a century and a half'.[2]

In a similar way, when Dronsfield introduces 'Madame Beswick' and her haunted granary, he implies this is a *known* local legend, that knowledge of Madame Beswick's story has continued to be passed down in her hometown, even if it had been forgotten by the Manchester Natural History Society and its visitors.

This is borne out by some responses to Dronsfield's story, such as a letter to the *Manchester Guardian* in 1877 that summarises Dronsfield's piece and asserts that 'tradition affords' that Madame Beswick lived at Birchen Bower, Hollinwood.[3]

In many ways, it is impossible to separate the author of the story from its location. There has been very little biography written about James Dronsfield – even in comparison to his collaborators, Brierley and Bamford – and the most significant detail preserved about his life and career is the fact that he came from Hollinwood. As this was a place that, from 1869, would be a canonical element of the Manchester Mummy story, some information on the place is required in order to understand both the author and the content of the 'Legend of Birchen Bower'.

Oldham was – and is – a town a few miles north-east of Manchester, close to the Pennines and served by the rivers Irk and Medlock. The Metropolitan Borough of Oldham takes in both the town of Oldham and numerous smaller towns and villages (from Chadderton and Failsworth in the west, to Saddleworth in the east, itself a conglomeration of villages and hamlets), but this configuration was not put in place until the Local Government Act 1972 and the creation of Greater Manchester. At the time James Dronsfield was writing, all of these towns and villages were separate entities, trying to avoid being subsumed into their two larger neighbours, Oldham and Manchester.[4]

Hollinwood was traditionally an area of Chadderton, a manorial township in the historic country of Lancashire, whose landlords included the powerful families of Radclyffe, Assheton (or Ashton), Chetham and Trafford. Chadderton had two post-medieval manor houses: Chadderton Hall (built by the de Chaddertons but owned by the Ashtons for centuries) and Foxdenton Hall (owned by the Radclyffes). It was a wealthy town, surrounded by farmland and countryside, which became only wealthier with the industrial revolution. By the 1920s, Chadderton boasted an Urban District Council, a grand town hall, a Carnegie library and a public swimming baths. By the 1930s, it was the second most populous urban district in the country, and it started the process of obtaining municipal borough status, though these ambitions were thwarted by a downturn in the town's prosperity in part caused by the Great Depression, and in part due to the collapse of the local coal mining industry.

When Dronsfield was writing, Chadderton was just entering its most prosperous phase, having joined the cotton business later than Manchester and Oldham but with just as much gusto, but also (like its close neighbour Failsworth) having the lucrative silk-weaving and hat-making sectors to augment its cotton mills. It's no surprise, then, to see Dronsfield calling back to more rural times in his writing, as an attempt to capture 'Lancashire character' that both pre-dates and survives the mills and factories that were starting to dominate.

Hollinwood, a village on the border of Chadderton and Failsworth, survived as farmland and countryside longer than Chadderton itself. Its name suggests an origin as moorland or common, where holly (hollin) grew.[5] The Ordnance Survey map published in 1882 (surveyed in 1844–63) shows an area that is almost entirely fields, with some small clusters of buildings around the 'New Road' (now part of the A62 between Oldham and Manchester). Birchen Bower appears on this map as farmland accessed from an area called Bradley Bent along Bower Lane, but bounded on one side by the Rochdale Canal (opened in 1804) and the Birchen Bower Rope Mills on the other.

This is the place that Dronsfield is trying to capture in his writing, an area that is still 'traditionally Lancashire' but clearly under threat from the gentle but inexorable encroachment of canals and mills. It is also a small, insignificant village that no one will have heard of, and so to publish a 'legend' of the place is to give it gravitas, tradition and identity.

Although it's not possible to verify Dronsfield's claims that the legend of Madame Beswick was well known in the local area prior to his publishing it in 1869 – while some people claimed to know the story, their verification only appeared *after* it was published – some elements of it accord with other evidence or anecdote. For instance, it appears other stories circulated about local people's fears around the approach of Bonnie Prince Charlie's army, such as the claim that the farmers of Shelderslow in Springhead hid their cattle in nearby woodland to protect them from the Jacobite invasion.[6] And the descriptions of Birchen Bower as being secluded and nestled in woodland is plausible given its name – Birchen referring to birch trees – and the fact that Hollinwood Chapel was built using timber from the woodlands of Birchen Bower in the 1760s.[7]

Nevertheless, other elements of Dronsfield story read more like myth, such as the reports of supernatural occurrences at the barn, and are perhaps psychologically implausible. No explanation is given, for instance, as to why Madame Beswick didn't retrieve her hidden treasure once the immediate threat of Jacobite invasion had passed or why that then translated into a desire to prevent her family members from inheriting after her death.

* * *

Dronsfield's story was significant, creating an Oldham (or Chadderton) legend out of a Manchester curiosity. In localizing the story to Madame Beswick's alleged home in Hollinwood, it transformed the story into a piece of Oldham folklore and, to an extent, it remains such today. While Miss Beswick is often called 'the Manchester Mummy', she is also called 'the mummy of Birchen Bower', and the story is still considered a 'local' one in Hollinwood and Failsworth.

However, Dronsfield's account found a life outside of Oldham, and among readers and writers entirely unfamiliar with Hollinwood and its environs. For these writers, the romantic name of 'Birchen Bower' was enough to conjure a particular environment and setting for a decidedly curious ghost story.

John H. Ingram's book *The Haunted Homes and Family Traditions of Great Britain* was published in 1897, and it includes a version of the Madame Beswick story. Ingram states that his version of the story is 'derived chiefly' from Dronsfield's 1869 article, and largely follows the plot laid out by his predecessor.

Stating outright that 'gold is at the bottom of the story', Ingram explains that 'old Miss Beswick' (who he has explained was buried at Harpurhey Cemetery after her stint in the Natural History Museum) was 'crafty' and ensured that the 'rightful heirs of Birchen Bower, Rose Hill and Cheetwood Estates' were denied their inheritance by her 'stratagem'. Birchen Bower, he explains, was an 'ancient homestead', 'a quaint four-gabled edifice, built in the form of a cross, and remarkable for the beauty of its summer surroundings'.[8] After recounting the story of the buried treasure and its discovery by Joe at Tamer's, Ingram turns his attention to the continued haunting of Birchen Bower by its former occupant:

> Madame Beswick, indeed, still haunts the old neighbourhood; on clear, moonlight [*sic*] nights she walks in a headless state between the old barn and the horsepool, and at other times assumes the forms of different animals, but is always lost sight of near the horsepool: this causes some folk to fancy that she concealed something there during the Scottish invasion, which she is now desirous of pointing out to anyone courageous enough to speak to her.[9]

I have to interject briefly to draw attention to the fact that the ghost of Madame Beswick is, here, 'headless'. Not only does this detail make no sense, given that at no point in her afterlife as a mummy was Miss Beswick's head removed – indeed, most accounts draw attention to the fact that her face was visible, definitely suggesting her head was still attached – it also contradicts Ingram's own account, which earlier had described the ghost of Madame Beswick appearing to a local 'rustic' in the dusk with 'streams of blue light seeming to dart from her eyes and flash on the horror-stricken man'.[10]

Returning to Ingram's account of the continued haunting of Birchen Bower:

> On dark and dreary winter nights the barn, it is said, appears to be on fire; a red glare of glowing heat being observable through the loop-holes and crevices of the building, and strange, unearthly noises proceed from it, as if Satan and all his imps were holding jubilee there. Sometimes, indeed, the sight is so threatening that the neighbours will raise an alarm and knock up the farmer and tell him the barn is in flames. When the premises are searched, however, nothing is found wrong, everything is in order, and the neighbours go terror-stricken home, fully convinced that they have witnessed another of Madame Beswick's supernatural pranks.[11]

As noted, Ingram is clear that his account is 'derived chiefly' from Dronsfield's. The problem is that the two stories were published thirty years apart. By 1897, Ingram's description of haunted Hollinwood doesn't ring true at all.

Between Dronsfield's account and Ingram's book, the Lancashire and Yorkshire Railway had opened its Thorpes Bridge to Oldham Werneth line, which was completed in 1880 and cut across the land in between the 'new road' (now Oldham Road) and what had been Birchen Bower. On 1 April 1881, Hollinwood Station opened on this line, sitting on the corner of Bower Lane and the newly constructed Railway Road. Several fields around Birchen Bower were turned over to mining and the construction of the Bower Colliery, which would in turn be sold to Ferranti's, an electrical engineering company, in 1896. A tramway was constructed between the Rochdale Canal and the Bower Colliery, though this seems to have been removed prior to the construction of the Ferranti factory at the end of the 1890s. If an old barn did survive all of this, and if its owner (unlikely to be a farmer at this point) did see 'a red glare of glowing heat' and hear 'strange, unearthly noises', would it not be more likely he would attribute the Satanic jubilee to the railway, the tramway or the coalpit rather than 'Madame Beswick's supernatural pranks'?

If this sounds like conjecture, it's actually based on my experience of how the story is understood and passed on in and around Hollinwood itself in the present day. The Ferranti factory is a cornerstone of Hollinwood local history, and although the factory closed decades ago, it's still within living memory and was a major employer. When I've spoken about the Hannah Beswick story to local history and community groups in Hollinwood and Failsworth, not only is the story generally known, but the geography is navigated with reference to Ferranti's, the factory recreation ground (which was called 'The Bower' and is now the site of a Morrison's supermarket) and the railway station (now Hollinwood Metrolink stop). I have no doubt that residents of Hollinwood in 1897 would have used a similar set of landmarks to understand the story, and so could only have read Ingram's story as a description of past, rather than present, hauntings.

But for readers outside Hollinwood, these landmarks would play no part in their reception of the story, and so they might easily believe that Birchen Bower continued to exist in rural, ghostly seclusion.

Around the same time as Ingram's book was published, an alternative version of the story appeared. Henry Frith, an Irish engineer, translator and prolific author, published a book entitled *Haunted Ancestral Homes: True Ghost Stories* at some point in the 1890s. The original publication details for the book are now lost, but a self-published ebook edition appeared on Lulu in 2017, in which the editor claims a date of 1892.[12] Certainly, Frith's book came out before 1902, as it was serialized in newspapers at this point. In the absence of an original edition of Frith's book, I'm going to use the text as printed in the *Ripon Observer*, January 1902, as this appears to be the fullest available version of the text and includes quite a lot of material that isn't found in the 2017 ebook, including the claim at the end of the story that '[m]any of the particulars appeared in an Oldham paper several years ago', linking it back to Dronsfield's account.[13]

Frith's take on the story is titled, 'The Buried Treasure of Birchen Bower; or, the Headless Seeker', and it begins:

> A dismal autumn evening. The mist hangs heavy on the silent landscape, and wreaths in ghostly folds above the stream. Along the highway

> rides carefully a man of sober garb and mien, who, passing the ancient Bower House, continues his way to a smaller residence by the river side of Birchen, Lancashire.[14]

Frith's account is heavy on pathetic fallacy, but light on local geography, with 'Birchen' being understood as both the place name and a river appearing across the fields.

The 'man of sober garb and mien' turns out to be a Dr White, riding through the mists to visit an elderly patient. He approaches an isolated house:

> The old gabled mansion, even then falling to delay, was slowly swallowed up in the swirling mist, now agitated by an almost imperceptible breeze, which hardly stirred the dying leaves on the trees, or deflected from their course those that fell fluttering to the ground.[15]

But this is not the house to which the doctor is travelling. He goes past the decaying mansion to a smaller house nearby, knocks on the door, and is greeted by an elderly servant called Bridget. He then goes to speak, in secret, with Bridget's mistress, the equally elderly Miss Beswick:

> The old lady, Miss Beswick, had, in former days, in the stirring times of the 'Forty Five', resided in her house – the old Bower House aforementioned. But nervous fears of the Pretender and his adherents, the dread of plunder, the lonely situation, and the natural nervous temperament, induced the lady to quit her house, and to reside in a smaller one, where she was not so liable to be robbed, as she thought. The assailants might work their wicked will upon the old house – they would not find her treasured hoards or hoarded treasure! Not they. It was all too securely hidden.
>
> But old age increased; and as the time approached when the ageing spinster knew that in all probability she must leave this sphere, and pass into the unknown, she became more and more imbued with the fear of dissolution. 'Earth to earth – dust to dust,' was a sentence she had a horror of. Was her body, still well-shapen and not uncomely for her years, to be resolved into dust in the grave? She could not bear the idea of being buried, and of crumbling then to decay.
>
> By degrees her mind became so imbued with this spirit of resistance to the final sentence on humanity, that she made up her mind to avoid it. Her body should never be buried, her spirit should not forsake the place where all her wealth and her hopes in life were centred. Her body

> must remain in possession, even if the estate must pass to strangers or relatives.[16]

Frith's version of the story follows the plot of Dronsfield's account, but with romantic dramatization. The character of Bridget is new, but she turns out to be the aunt of Joe at Tamer's (now Joe, who works at Tanner's Mills) who discovers the gold at Birchen Bower and takes it to St Ann's Square to be exchanged for cash. The rest of the account is fairly similar to Ingram's in its descriptions of subsequent hauntings, though Frith is more condemnatory about the role of the doctor, claiming that he colluded with Miss Beswick to deprive her relatives of their inheritance and ended up claiming the estate for himself. And while Ingram states that the haunting of Birchen Bower continues to this day, Frith is more careful to use the past tense for the barn haunting and Satanic jubilee episodes. He muses on whether the hauntings were supposed to end with the burial of her body, the death of Dr White, the discovery of her treasure, or the reinstatement of the true heirs of Birchen Bower:

> It would be interesting to learn whether anyone has very lately seen the elderly lady whose headless spirit has for so many years haunted the old house at Hollingwood [*sic*]. Whether the interment which took place in 1868 has restored the property to the relatives of the deceased lady only local lawyers can tell. At any rate, the body was embalmed, the gold was found, and there have not been lacking many witnesses to the apparition of Birchen Bower House.[17]

Interestingly, Frith also offers a suggestion around the relationship between the Peter Street Mummy and the Legend of Birchen Bower that does seem to fit with the sequence of events outlined so far (supernatural element aside). When he reaches his description of the burial – which he, like Ingram, quotes from the *Manchester Guardian* report of August 1868 – he writes:

> This ceremony was accordingly performed on the 22nd of July, 1868, and aroused some curiosity. What was this body which was thus quietly interred? Whose was it? The deceased doctor had placed it in his museum, no doubt, but for what reason?
>
> Inquiry was made, and, of course, the incident reached the local papers. The old stories were revived, and no doubt certain incidents and items of information were added.[18]

I have to agree with Frith's assessment here. It does seem like certain items of information – like a Satanic jubilee and a ghost that shoots bolts of blue light from its eyes – were definitely added to the story.

* * *

On a more serious note, the effect of this 'revival' of the 'old stories' about Madame Beswick and her buried treasure added items of biographical information that would have an impact on both the reception of the Manchester Mummy story and an understanding of the character of Miss Beswick.

It's clear from Dronsfield's account and those that followed that the story of Madame Beswick's buried treasure revolves around the idea of disinheritance, keeping 'rightful' heirs from property and riches that 'should' be theirs. In these versions, Miss Beswick is an 'eccentric testatrix', but rather than coming from superstition or phobia, this is the result of miserliness, greed or even downright cruelty, with the restoration of the 'true' inheritors of Birchen Bower only coming when her body was buried at Harpurhey (though Frith doubts whether even that resolved the issue).

The question of the woman's will would resurface on occasion with more serious scrutiny, with correspondents to local newspapers throwing doubt on the alleged document's validity. As Dronsfield's article had provided enough biographical information to identify 'Madame Beswick', even people with no local connection or memory of the story were able to piece together information about her, including finally getting the answers to the questions that had vexed Robert Dukinfield Darbishire: the woman's Christian name (Hannah) and the date of her will (1758). Research could also easily reveal the names of various properties owned by her family and the (apparent) names of her brothers, John and Wright. And, as English law states that a will becomes a public document once a grant of probate is issued, it was now also possible to track down the woman's will and find out what her final wishes actually were.

Questions about the possibility of legal impropriety hovered around the edges of the story for some time – in fact, it's possible to find more recent accounts that imply some level of uncertainty around the terms of Miss Beswick's will. In the immediate aftermath of Dronsfield's article, this uncertainty is raised as 'polite scrutiny' or 'public interest'. For instance, a letter in the *Middleton Guardian* in June 1889 asked:

> Can any of your readers give any information respecting the family of Miss Hannah Beswick, who died at her residence in Cheetwood-lane, now known as Cheetwood Old Hall, in the year 1758. She left considerable property in various localities, amongst which were the house and lands in Cheetwood, messuages, tenements, &c., called by the names of 'Claytons' and 'Bradley Bent', at Chadderton; and also 'Birchen Bower', at Hollinwood [...] I should like to have all the details possible of this lady's family, particularly in respect to her father and brothers and any of their descendants.[19]

While this might be innocent scholarly research, the final question about her father, brothers and possible descendants does look more like a query over inheritance than anything else. A response appeared in the paper the following month:

> The name of the father of Miss Hannah Beswick was John – his sons were John and Wright. At Birchen Bower Farm, Hollinwood (near the station), over the barn door, is inscribed 'I.B., 1728', the 'I' being the initial for John. The sons never married, and at their deaths their sister (Miss Beswick) became heiress to the whole of the extensive properties in this and other counties. The Robinson family inherited the main of the property. Several families about Oldham, Hyde, and elsewhere claim relationship, if not heirship, to this notable family, and can doubtless give a concise history of same, if needed for any useful purpose.[20]

Here is the barn from the ghost story versions of the story (located 'near the station', which opened eight years prior to the letter being written) but translated from a site of 'supernatural pranks' to a material testimony to family history. This might serve, the letter-writer coyly suggests, a 'useful purpose', as there are families in the area who might 'claim relationship, if not heirship'.

The letter I previously quoted from 1877, in which the writer (called Mary Malin) claims to remember the 'traditions' of Miss Beswick's hidden treasure, also includes a claim of disinheritance: 'One story is that a brother who lived at the farm displeased her by cutting down a favourite willow tree, and she therefore arranged matters so that none of her fortune should fall into his hands.'[21] And, as it was now possible (if one looked carefully) to determine that Hannah Beswick's brother John predeceased her (by either twenty-one or twelve years, depending which John Beswick you had found), the most common line of enquiry was the younger brother, Wright Beswick.[22] While some, like the respondent in the *Middleton Guardian* of 1889, claimed that Wright had also predeceased his sister, this fact was far from certain. Mary Malin's account of the willow tree disinheritance implies that the brother outlived the sister, and this came to be the dominant story.

So insistent was the belief that the descendants of Wright Beswick had been denied their inheritance or, at the very least, had been denied the right to bury their relative with a more appropriate funeral than the one organized by the Commissioners of the Natural History Society, that even the cemetery in which Miss Beswick was buried began to get cold feet about the legitimacy of it all. In December 1889, an advertisement appeared in newspapers across the north-west of England: 'TO PARISH CLERKS AND OTHERS – FIVE POUNDS will be GIVEN for the CERTIFICATE of Baptism, or Marriage, of WRIGHT, the son of JOHN BESWICK, of Birchen Bower. He was born 1705. REGISTRAR, Harpurhey Cemetery, Manchester.'[23] I have been unable to find out whether any parish clerk claimed his five pounds.

Early in the twentieth century, the local historian H. T. Crofton – who claimed to have seen the body of Hannah Beswick many times when it was displayed in the museum – wrote to the *Manchester City News* to dispel some myths about the case, but he ended up adding fuel to the 'eccentric testatrix' fire:

> Since the days of De Quincey, at least, a legend of which there were many slightly varying forms, has been current in Manchester, the most coherent version of which ran that good old Dr Charles White received £25,000 under the will of Miss Hannah Beswick of Cheetwood, who died in 1757, on condition that he kept her body above ground for one hundred years. She had had a relative nearly buried alive. He was to take a veil from her face periodically in the presence of witnesses [...] Recently a relative denied this tale, but recorded another which most unworthily reflected on the doctor's integrity. This fiction was that the doctor was the executor, and received a legacy of £400 to pay funeral expenses and to distribute any surplus amongst Miss Beswick's relatives, but to avoid any funeral expense he embalmed the body and so pocketed the whole

> legacy. As the first myth was very incredible and the second was monstrous, it seemed worth while to try and lay the ghost, or both ghosts, by referring to the will. It was proved at Chester, and is very lengthy, but Mr W.F. Irvine, who has kindly examined it for me, says there is not a word in it about embalming, nor was Dr White an executor, and he merely received a legacy of £100, while the £400 was left, not to him, but to the executrices, Mary Creeme and Esther Robinson 'in order to defray the expenses of my funeral, and if there be any overplus to dispose of the same discretionally among my father's relations, &c., without giving account to any person, &c., for all or any part'. The will mentions many beneficiaries named Robinson, and it is endorsed with a memorandum relating to a lawsuit.[24]

Crofton is keen to debunk certain myths here, offering hard evidence of their falsity. Except, the evidence is only partial and second-hand, as Crofton reveals that, even though the will is a public document, it isn't the sort of thing you can easily peruse. It is lengthy, located in an archive outside Manchester, and, though he doesn't say it, it is written in eighteenth-century legal language and handwriting. He has relied on Mr W. F. Irvine (presumably an archivist) to give him the salient points. He also mentions a 'relative' who has denied Thomas de Quincey's account of the embalming and suggested instead some foul play about inheritance (though he doesn't say who this relative is). When he debunks *that* story, he offers the will as evidence, and notes at the end that there has been 'a lawsuit' related to the will – but he gives no details as to what that related to or how it was resolved. The will of Hannah Beswick remains an uncertain, legally dubious document, even when cited as 'fact'.

It might have become apparent from these various tellings and retellings of the story that the location of Birchen Bower comes in and out of view. While some writers have Birchen Bower as the home of Hannah Beswick, others (like Crofton) give her address as Cheetwood, and others list a number of properties including both Cheetwood and Birchen Bower among others.

Cheetwood is an area at the northern edge of Manchester, around five miles from Hollinwood, and I'll be exploring its role in the story in the next chapter. For now, I want to introduce a final location: Sale Priory, a house situated in the historic county of Cheshire, around six miles south-west of Manchester. In 1931, when this house was scheduled for demolition, it was also claimed as the location for Hannah Beswick's buried treasure:

> Treasure Hunt at Doomed Priory
> Owner Who Was Unburied for 100 Years
> A hunt for a treasure buried 185 years ago in Sale Priory, near Manchester, is to be made shortly when the local council starts to demolish the buildings.
> The treasure was the property of Miss Hannah Beswick, a wealthy Manchester woman, who died over 100 years ago, and who once owned the Priory.
> In 1745, when rebels appeared in the neighbourhood, she buried it and never revealed its hiding place.
> Now Mr C.H. Megson, of Sale, whose father lived at the Priory until 1921, has asked Sale Council, on behalf of the Priory trustees, to hunt for the treasure when the building is demolished.
> By her own wish, Miss Beswick was not buried until 100 years had elapsed after her death.[25]

Even in the twentieth century, with a will that, as H. T. Crofton pointed out, can be read, at least in abstracted form, and, as James Dronsfield claimed, 'local legends' of her life in Hollinwood being well known in the area, the story of Hannah Beswick wasn't pinned definitively to a particular location.

Sale Priory and Mr C. H. Megson will also return in the next chapter, but I quote the 1931 story to show how pernicious the idea of the 'buried treasure' and disinheritance was. It may be that the idea was so romantic – particularly when it included the possibility of a 'treasure hunt' (like Mr C. H. Megson wished to see) or a chance discovery (like that of Joe at Tamer's) – that it was hard to resist including it in the more poetic retellings of the legend.

However, when coupled with the continued raising of 'heirship', 'rightful heirs', the search for the descendants of Wright Beswick and the enigmatic 'lawsuit' relating to Hannah Beswick's will, it all feels more like a question mark over the legality of the woman's will. The more romanticized versions of the story, in which the woman is driven by cruel miserliness, revenge over a perceived slight, or pathological superstition leaves us wondering whether this is something more than an 'eccentric testatrix'. Was Hannah Beswick of sound mind? Was she coerced into writing a will that favoured her doctor? Are there legal improprieties about the properties? Did she even have the right to decide what to do with these properties?

Although earlier reports of the Manchester Mummy had introduced the idea of the 'eccentric testatrix', this was without any suggestion that her final wishes should not be honoured. The 'Legend of Birchen Bower' casts doubt on this, with the supernatural and romanticized elements creating an atmosphere of mystery in which there *must* be something dubious going on. As we have seen, this led to infrequent, but repeated, suggestions that the will or the ownership of property was to be challenged, and the search was on for Wright Beswick, a more appropriate male line through which Cheetwood, Birchen Bower and the other estates could descend … even if he did kill his sister's favourite willow tree.

6
Tinned salmon

In July 1890, a shocking story appeared in Manchester's local newspapers. The *Middleton Guardian* gave it the headline 'A Ghastly Find at Cheetham', and other papers went with similar phrases. The story began:

> Two labourers, named John Fogg and John Clark, who are employed at a brickworks off Derby-street, Cheetham, made a dreadful discovery while following their employment on Tuesday morning. The works are situated in the middle of a plot of vacant land which is bounded on one side by Derby-street and on another side by the high wall which runs along the rear of Strangeways Prison. In the course of the operations at the brickworks it was found necessary, in order to maintain the supply of clay, to pull down Cheetwood Hall, an ancient building which at one time was a picturesque landmark [...] The old structure, with its latticed windows and timber supports, was, as we have stated, demolished so that its site might yield material for the brick makers. Clay getting went on uneventfully until Tuesday morning, when the two workmen made a discovery of a startling character. While digging away at a depth of four or five feet from what once was the ground floor of the old hall they met with an obstruction. It turned out to be a wooden coffin of medium length. With some difficulty they succeeded in recovering it from the clay in which it was firmly embedded, and proceeding further in their investigations, they opened the shell to find inside an oblong leaden box. On the box being opened it was seen to contain what are believed to be human remains, although as yet no definite opinion can be expressed upon the point. The appearance they presented is described as tinned salmon, and one strange and unaccountable circumstance is that no bones were seen. It should be stated, however, that only a cursory examination was made, one probable reason for which is that the stench which issued from the box when it was opened was almost overpowering. Although the coffin

> was of medium size, the leaden box in which the supposed remains were found is not more than four feet in length, and its shape does not bear any resemblance to the cases which are usually prepared for the reception of human remains.[1]

The story went on to outline how Fogg and Clark disagreed about which part of Cheetwood Hall would have stood over their ghastly find, with one suggesting it was the sitting room and the other the entrance hall. The article then raised the spectre of Hannah Beswick, quoting a 'Prestwich correspondent' who pointed out that the hall was the former residence of the 'Manchester mummy' and was 'for some time the resting place of her remains after embalmment by Doctor Charles White in 1758'. The unnamed correspondent goes on to suggest some theories as to the meaning of the 'ghastly find':

> Whose remains are those now unearthed, and why were they so disposed of? Is it possible that the coffin contains the corpse of the said Miss Beswick, and that the reputed 'mummy' was simply a make-up and make-believe for some reason or other? It is notorious that Miss Beswick's mother, 'Patience' (whose husband, John, died in 1705), disappeared, no one knows how; and it is suggested that she may have met with foul play, and that the remains now found may be hers.[2]

These suggestions are contradicted by an interview with Superintendent Godby of the City Police's B Division, who explains that:

> [T]he house was formerly occupied by a Dr White, who lived there for many years in the old 'body snatching' days when considerable difficulty was experienced in securing bodies for dissection. From the appearance of the contents of the coffin and the absence of skull or bones, he has come to the conclusion that they are portions of bodies which have been taken to a doctor's house for the purpose of dissection. Supposing murder had been committed, he pointed out that would certainly have been found the remains of both skull and bones.[3]

And a final correspondent, giving their address as Halliwell-lane, adds:

> The information given clearly establishes the suggestion that had been made that the remains found in the coffin consisted of only portions of the body of Hannah Beswick, which were taken out by Dr White preparatory to the embalmment. The doctor was one of her trustees. The deceased lady left in her will a sum of £400 to defray the expenses of her funeral, and her executors were instructed to hand over any surplus, if there should be any remaining, to her father's relatives, but distinctly

> stated that her executors were not to be questioned or held accountable for the manner in which the money was spent. The executors were Mary Greame and Esther Robinson. This undoubtedly suggests that a secret arrangement was made by her with the doctor to keep her body unburied for a specified time, as it is reported that she had a great fear of being buried alive. It would be an act of decency and a respectful recognition to the descendants of the deceased lady if the remains were placed with the embalmed trunk of Miss Beswick, which was interred in Harpurhey Cemetery in 1868, 110 years after her decease.[4]

The *Middleton Guardian*'s resumé of the commentary on the 'ghastly find' reads like a Manchester Mummy Choose Your Own Adventure. It's got murder, body-snatching, taphophobia, an eccentric testatrix and a museum hoax.

Even more commentary appeared in other newspapers, with a correspondent ('NO NAME') to the *Manchester Courier* casting sly aspersions on the Natural History Society:

> The remains just exhumed at Cheetwood being thought by many persons to form part of the corpse of Miss Hannah Beswick, I think the authorities would only be doing a decent thing by ordering the same to be interred in the grave which has held the other part of the said lady's anatomy (in the shape of the 'Manchester Mummy') since 1868. The grave of Miss Beswick, I understand, does not even boast a simple memorial stone notwithstanding by her will she left £400 for the purposes of her funeral. It would be interesting to learn from some source what became of the said funeral money, and, if available, whether a fitting memorial could not be erected over her resting place? I presume the Natural History Society who undertook the interment of the 'mummy' 110 years after the decease had no handling of the said handsome sum, seeing how they studied economy in the matter. Can any of your readers state briefly where the 'mummy' was located prior to its exhibition in the Manchester Natural History Museum?[5]

And a correspondent to the *Manchester Times* fleshed out (no pun intended) the story of the mysterious 'Patience':

> Miss Beswick was the daughter to John and Patience Beswick, of Cheetwood Old Hall, Manchester. John Beswick died in 1706, leaving two children, the said Hannah and John; another boy, Wright, was born four months after his decease. The relict, Patience, it is said, afterwards married a butcher, of Ashton-Under-Lyne, named Walker, who murdered her. Patience was a daughter of John Buckley, of Saddleworth. The

> residence of Miss Beswick was Birchen Bower, Hollinwood, Oldham, but the eminent Doctor Charles White (her physician, and one of her trustees) gave up to her the paternal home at Cheetwood, where she died. Can any of your readers give an authentic history of Miss Beswick's mother, Patience, and the posthumous child, Wright? It has never been satisfactorily explained why Dr White kept Miss Beswick's body above ground. Miss Beswick's will certainly gave no authority for such an unusual proceeding.[6]

The *Manchester Times* also noted that, while Superintendent Godby believed the remains to be 'portions of bodies which have been taken to a doctor's house for the purpose of dissection', Dr Dearden, the police surgeon who attended the scene with him, suggested otherwise, pointing out that dissection would leave the flesh in smaller fragments than those found in the lead box:

> The only explanation other than that just mentioned which Dr Dearden considers at all probable is that Dr White purchased a body with a view of obtaining a skeleton, and removed the flesh in large pieces, which he afterwards buried to avoid any awkward questions. Against this theory, however, there is the fact that the oak coffin is evidently the work of a professional coffinmaker and is bent in the usual manner – a very unlikely receptacle for the flesh of some chance subject of the 'body-snatchers' craft. The suggestion of foul play does not seem to receive any support, but the whole affair remains decidedly mysterious.[7]

If James Dronsfield's article in the *Oldham Weekly Chronicle* served to transform the story of the Manchester Mummy into a ghost story, the 'Ghastly Find at Cheetham' turned it into an urban legend.

* * *

In his influential work on urban legends, *The Vanishing Hitchhiker*, Jan Harold Brunvand explores a definition and understanding of 'urban legends', a specific and modern form of narrative folklore, that continues to inform both academic articles and more popular writing on the form. He outlines certain elements that are common to urban legends: they are 'told seriously, circulate largely by word of mouth, are generally anonymous, and vary constantly in particular details from one telling to another, while always preserving a central core of traditional elements or "motifs"'. In addition to this, there is 'usually no geographical or generational gap between teller and event'; an urban legend 'is *true*', it 'really occurred, and recently, and always to someone else who is quite close to the narrator, or at least "a friend of a friend"'. Significantly, urban legends are 'a unique, unselfconscious reflection of major concerns of individuals in the societies in which the legends circulate'.[8]

As has been clear from the various accounts of the Hannah Beswick story I've explored so far, the story *is* generally 'told seriously' but in versions that 'vary constantly in particular details from one telling to another'. The frequent use of phrases such as 'it is said' and 'so the story runs' imply a word-of-mouth circulation, and the surfacing of details in 1890 that hadn't previously appeared in printed versions of the story seems to confirm this. The question is, can we really say that the story of Hannah Beswick contains the other important elements of an urban legend: the 'friend of a friend' appeal to authority and the 'unconscious reflection of major concerns'?

Let's start with the 'friend of a friend'.

It obviously isn't true to say that there is no 'generational gap between teller and event' in the case of the Hannah Beswick story, as accounts always rely on the fact that it happened many years ago, usually outside of living memory. However, it is possible to discern a tendency towards closing that gap in some tellings, specifically those in which the teller claims a personal connection to the narrative.

After the 'Ghastly Find at Cheetham' story appeared in the local press, a man named George Beswick wrote to the *Manchester Times* claiming that Hannah Beswick was his grandfather's niece (and so his second cousin), and that there were questions related to her will and the ownership of a certain (unnamed) piece of property that his family were intending to resolve. A response to the letter from a J. Davenport of Prestwich pointed out that the close family relationship claimed by George Beswick was an 'anachronism', given that the man claimed his grandfather died in 1866, and yet the supposed niece died in 1758. This response also asked for George Beswick to supply the name of the property in dispute and give details of the 'Manchester gentleman' who allegedly had plans of the estate to support the challenge to the will.[9] George Beswick wrote back to say that he couldn't answer those questions, and that perhaps he'd misunderstood the relationship between Hannah Beswick and himself.

George Beswick wasn't the first person to claim a family relationship to Hannah Beswick, and he certainly wouldn't be the last. In the previous chapter, I quoted letter from a woman named Mary Malin that appeared in the *Manchester Guardian*. In this letter, Mary Malin claimed that 'Madame Beswick was a kinswoman of my mother', and that the story had been 'narrated from childhood in [her] family'. Mary Malin recounts the story included in James Dronsfield's 1869 article, and her own version of the story doesn't deviate from the 'central core' but instead embellishes it with small details, such as Madame Beswick's request to have her body placed 'in her own summer-house, in a coffin with glass at the top', and that there was 'a trial with respect to a portion of her property, over 50 years ago'.[10]

Mary Malin's story appeared before George Beswick's, but both include the detail of a dispute about Hannah Beswick's will, as well as a half-remembered family relationship to the woman herself. Mary Malin's claim to proximity – 'a kinswoman of my mother' – is both vague enough to withstand scrutiny (unlike George Beswick's) and close enough to confer authority on her version of the story. It implies, perhaps, that Madame Beswick was of the same generation as Mary Malin's mother, which would be an 'anachronism' but would serve to close the 'generational gap'. 'Kinswoman of my mother' isn't so different to 'friend of a friend'.

Where a family relationship cannot be claimed, or where it isn't possible to close the 'generational gap', the 'geographical gap' is the focus of attention. There is a long and continuing history of people claiming a connection to either the location of the Hannah Beswick story or some material artefact associated with the woman. In a previous chapter, we saw an early example of this, when Mr Browne-Clayton (or someone connected to him) claimed to have a 'coffin intended for Miss Beswick' in his stable. Once the 'facts' of Hannah Beswick's identity, and that of Dr White, were revealed in the popular press, Mr Browne-Clayton's story ceased to make much sense, given that the man didn't live in any of the properties associated with the woman's story. Nevertheless, the coffin itself would reappear in other tellings of the story.

* * *

The 'Mummy of Birchen Bower' and the 'Ghastly Find at Cheetham' might offer very different versions of the Hannah Beswick story, but they do have one important thing in common – they attach the story to a very particular location, localizing the 'Manchester Mummy' to Hollinwood and Cheetwood respectively. At the beginning of the twentieth century, another location would start to appear as the site of the Hannah Beswick story.

In 1903, Herbert W. Smith wrote an account of the story in *Manchester Faces and Places*. In his narration of the story, Smith asserts that the body of Hannah Beswick was embalmed, not at Cheetwood Old Hall as had been claimed in 1890, but at Sale Priory, the home of Charles White.

The Priory was a Georgian house – never actually a religious building – built in Sale, around six miles south-west of the centre of Manchester, by Thomas White, a Manchester lawyer and the grandfather of Dr Charles White. The house has now been demolished, with only the small woodland area known as Priory Gardens remaining as a reminder of the former residence. However, in 1903, when Smith wrote his account, the house was not only still standing, it was still occupied.

The version of the story that appeared in *Manchester Faces and Places* included a number of details familiar from earlier versions, though as might be expected, there were some embellishments. It states that a man named John Beswick had three children: 'Of these children two, John and Wright, were sons, and one, Hannah the subject of our enquiry – a daughter born in 1688, exactly twenty two years after the Great Fire of London.'[11] This daughter is presented, not as eccentric, but as vulnerable to the predations of fortune-hunters:

> Maiden ladies of means are not infrequently pursued by unscrupulous associates. Miss Beswick's medical attendant and, as afterwards transpired, her executor, was Dr Charles White, presumably a physician of some eminence, seeing that he owned two houses: one in King Street, Manchester; the other Cheetwood Hall in the neighbourhood.[12]

Smith connects Cheetwood Hall to Charles White – as some of the 1890 retellings had done – but Hannah Beswick, it seems, was the resident of Sale Priory. The article actually starts with a description of a curious feature of Sale Priory: 'For upwards of thirty years there rested upon the flat, leaded part of the roof, a leaded shell. Inside the leaden shell was a large oak coffin and inside the coffin reposed an enbalmed [*sic*] corpse.'[13] This appears to be a reversed image of the Ghastly Find, a lead box with a coffin inside, rather than a coffin with a lead box inside. It is also a reversed image of Mr Browne-Clayton's coffin-in-the-stable, as it appears the coffin *was* used to house the body of Hannah Beswick, albeit on the roof of a Georgian house rather than buried in a cemetery.

Smith's account then goes on to explain (sort of) how this coffin came to be kept on the roof of the house:

> Leaving £400 for funeral expenses, Dr White as executor was instructed to divide the surplus among the Beswick family, the bulk of the property being willed to her relations on the mother's side [...] Eighteen years after the embalming process, in 1776 Dr White 'shuffled off this mortal coil' leaving the mummy to its fate. Nobody claimed it. The roof of 'The Priory' continued to be its refuge [...] but the present occupant of 'The Priory' possesses the handles of the coffin once lodged on his roof. Twenty years ago, the coffin itself was in existence.[14]

While we might question why the coffin was kept, specifically, on the *roof* of the house, the importance of this article is that it affirms a material connection between the story of Hannah Beswick and Sale Priory. This, it seems, is the location of the apocryphal coffin (which may or may not be the same one as was kept in Mr Browne-Clayton's stable) and also the location in which the body was kept prior to it being deposited with the Manchester Natural History Society.

The story – strange as it might seem – has remained part of the local folklore of Sale, and I've heard anecdotally that some walking tours around the area still include the detail that Sale Priory was both Hannah Beswick's home and the location for her embalming and subsequent storage of her corpse. Obviously, this contradicts other versions of the story – both the long-standing association of Charles White with a property on King Street, and the 'Ghastly Find' story that located the embalming at Cheetwood Hall – but it still persists as an alternative geography of the story to this day. In 2016, a series of walking guides were produced for the Trafford borough of Greater Manchester (of which Sale is now part) as part of the Heritage Trees project, as a partnership between City of Trees, Transport for Greater Manchester and Trafford Strategic Sport & Physical Activity Partnership. The guide to 'Sale Water Park and Priory Gardens' – a 2.4-mile route 'designed to help you explore some of Trafford's most beautiful countryside and parks on foot' – included the following information: 'Priory Gardens: Once home to co-founder of Manchester Royal Infirmary Hospital, Dr Charles White (1728–1813) was also known for keeping the embalmed body of Hannah Beswick, the Manchester Mummy, on the roof of the Priory. The house was demolished in 1932.'[15]

The Heritage Trees walking guide followed in the footsteps of another pamphlet, published over one hundred years earlier, which also sought to market Sale Priory on the basis of its connection to Hannah Beswick. This pamphlet, simply entitled *Sale Priory* and illustrated with photographs of the house, included both the story of Hannah Beswick's taphophobia (ascribed here to the fact that 'her sister had had a narrow escape from being buried alive whilst in a trance') and an extract of what purports to be Hannah's father's will. It also includes a claim of authenticity, by reproducing the 'reminiscences' of a Mrs Hunter, née Williamson, 'whose people had held the Ashton Hall estate since 1600' (presumably referring to the estate in nearby Ashton-on-Mersey). Mrs Hunter's pedigree and the family's long-standing residence in the area gives the account authority and counteracts any potential unreliability implied by the word 'reminiscences'. Mrs Hunter states: 'The old part of the Priory was pulled down and it was made into a farm house and later into a residence and came into the possession of Miss Hannah Beswick. She planted many rare trees and is said to have brought the cedar from Mount Lebanon.'[16]

This account serves a similar purpose and uses similar strategies to the accounts of Hannah Beswick's life in Hollinwood given by James Dronsfield in the *Oldham Chronicle*. It humanizes the 'mummy' by giving a picture of the woman in life, rather than in death. It locates that life in a particular locale, and one which will be familiar to residents of the area at the time of writing. And it evokes the idea of a long-standing *local* memory of the woman, suggesting that people of the neighbourhood passed the story of her life down through the generations. In the case of the Sale story, the 'generational gap' is closed by the inclusion of the cedar tree. This tree could be viewed by visitors to the Priory in 1912, and yet it was allegedly planted by Hannah Beswick, collapsing the temporal distance between the modern visitor and the Manchester Mummy through the use of a material object.

If you find yourself wondering if the stories of Hannah Beswick at Sale Priory aren't just a little bit far-fetched, that the story of her travelling to Lebanon in pursuit of rare cedar trees is a bit fanciful, and the story of the body being kept on the roof of a house seems somewhat impractical, you are not the first person to have these doubts.

* * *

Ernest Bosdin Leech was born in Stretford, near Manchester, in 1875. After initially studying at Christ's College, Cambridge, he returned to Manchester and completed a degree in medicine in 1901, becoming an MD in 1907. He is now best remembered for his work at Manchester Royal Infirmary, where he was not only a physician but also one of the people responsible for the relocation of the hospital from Piccadilly Gardens in the centre of Manchester to a new site on Oxford Road. Bosdin Leech enters this story, however, in his capacity as president of the Manchester Medical Society, an office he took on in 1934.

As member, secretary and then president of the Manchester Medical Society, Bosdin Leech became fascinated by the history of medicine in Manchester, building up the society's archive and library into a substantial collection, which is now held in the University of Manchester's Special Collections. During this work, Bosdin Leech became familiar with the story of Hannah Beswick and her connection to Charles White – the co-founder of the hospital to which Bosdin Leech devoted much of his career. In 1934, one hundred years after the founding of the Manchester Medical Society, Bosdin Leech included the story of Hannah Beswick in his presidential address. The address was published and circulated, and the story of the Manchester Mummy once again caught the popular imagination with people writing to its author with their own information about the case.

The result of this was that Bosdin Leech became the second person to attempt to uncover the true story of Hannah Beswick, also known as the Manchester Mummy. And he got a lot further with it than Robert Dukinfield Darbishire had done, partly due to the fact that he at least knew the woman's Christian name and the date of her death. He was able to send off for a typed abstract of her will, which he received from the Lancashire Archives in July 1934. The archivist, Fred Booth, noted in the cover letter to the abstract that the will contradicted a number of the claims made about Hannah Beswick, not least that she left instructions about the preservation of her body after death, just as Mr W. F. Irvine had done when asked to examine the will on behalf of H. T. Crofton.[17]

Bosdin Leech also collected up ephemera and articles related to the Hannah Beswick story, and it is in his collection (now a university archive) that I was able to see the *Sale Priory* booklet of 1912 and the Smith article from *Manchester Faces and Places*. One of the enjoyable things about accessing these copies of the documents is that you get to see Bosdin Leech's own notes expressing his frustration about everything the accounts get wrong. On the Smith article, there is note stating: 'Much of this article seems to me erroneous or at any rate to require confirmation e.g. date of death of Chas. White is certainly wrong.'[18] And on another article, a story that appeared in the *Manchester Guardian* in April 1935 and claimed that Charles White hid the money from Hannah Beswick's bequest in the base of a stone monument at Sale Priory (according to 'local memory'), he wrote: 'So many errors in above that it is difficult to know how to refute them.'[19]

The article from the *Manchester Guardian* was sent to Bosdin Leech as a cutting. It seems that, after his presidential address of 1934, he became something of a go-to guy for all things Manchester Mummy. The cutting was originally sent to Dr E. M. Brockbank, another doctor at Manchester Royal Infirmary, who forwarded it on to his colleague to respond. The sender was Clarence Megson, and the cutting wasn't the only thing he sent.

Clarence Megson (aka Mr C. H. Megson who appeared in the previous chapter as a wannabe treasure hunter) was born in 1869, the son of Alfred H. Megson who was a member of Manchester City Council and, in the latter part of the nineteenth century, the tenant of Sale Priory.[20] In his letter to Brockbank, Clarence Megson explains that the Priory had indeed been the location for the storage of Hannah Beswick's body. Not only that, but he himself had seen the coffin in which her body was kept:

> When in May 1879 I went to live at the Priory the gardener acting as caretaker who had been there for very many years took me on the roof and showed me the place where the coffin used to be. The same day I saw the oak coffin burned and the handle was kept as a relic of the occasion.[21]

It's unfortunate that the *very day* Clarence Megson moved into the Priory, the coffin was destroyed, preventing any verification of its existence. However, the handle of the coffin remained in Megson's possession until the 1930s, when he offered it, along with the 1912 booklet on *Sale Priory*, to 'any museum of local interest'.[22] It's not clear whether any museum ever took him up on the offer, as the coffin handle doesn't resurface again after 1935. But it's important to note the call to authority in Megson's letter – not only is he claiming to have seen the coffin himself, but he offers testimony from 'the gardener acting as caretaker who had been there for very many years' to close the 'generational gap' and give the story authenticity.

Megson was not the only person to claim a connection to a material object related to the case. In 1934, after his presidential address, Bosdin Leech received a letter from J. Wilfrid Jackson, one of the curators at the Manchester Museum (the successor institution to the Natural History Society, built by Owens College, by then a constituent college of the Victoria University, and opened to the public in 1887). In his letter, Jackson states that the work table he used at the museum was the very table that was once used to store the body of Hannah Beswick at the Peter Street museum.[23]

Speaking of the old museum, which closed a little over sixty years before Bosdin Leech gave his presidential address to the Manchester Medical Society, it's not a surprise to find letters describing visits to see the Manchester Mummy when it was on display in the town. In November 1934, Wyndham Smith wrote to relate his story of visiting the mummy at the museum, and, in February 1949 (some sixteen years after Bosdin Leech first opened this can of worms) a Stephen C. Baxter wrote to say that his cousin, Mrs Gilbert Gorton, also saw the mummy at Peter Street.[24]

We'll return to Mrs Gilbert Gorton shortly, but in order to understand Bosdin Leech's correspondence with Stephen C. Baxter, we have to look at another letter from 1934.

Edward Rhodes wrote to Bosdin Leech in November 1934, claiming to be a descendant of the Beswick family. Unlike George Beswick and Mary Malin before him, Edward Rhodes was able to offer a family tree to support his claim.

Hannah Beswick was, according to Rhodes, born in 1698, the granddaughter of Charles and Sarah Beswick of Failsworth. Her father married a woman named Robinson and they had three children: John, Hannah and Wright. Wright Beswick went on to marry a woman named Charity Taylor of Chapel-en-le-Frith, and they had a son who they named John. This John Beswick – Hannah's nephew – married Patience Buckley of Shepton Mallet, and this is the line from which Edward Rhodes is descended.[25]

Bosdin Leech – in what some might call a rookie mistake at this point – took this genealogy at face value. It does seem to chime with some of the other information he'd been able to collect on the case, such as the abstract of Hannah Beswick's will, which leaves a number of bequests to cousins named Robinson. The reference to Hannah's grandparents coming from Failsworth also connects with the story of Birchen Bower, which was on the border of Chadderton and Failsworth.

So, when Stephen C. Baxter got in touch in 1949, Bosdin Leech believed he had an accurate family tree for Hannah Beswick.

Baxter's initial letter was sent to R. U. Sayce, Keeper of the Victoria Museum (i.e. the Manchester Museum). He says that he is writing a book, to be titled *Gorton of Gorton, Manchester*, and then explains the connection with the museum: 'Mrs Gilbert Gorton [his cousin] saw the mummy there many years ago, and states that Miss Beswick's mother was a Gorton before her marriage.'[26] Sayce, even after all that time, knew who to pass the letter to.

Bosdin Leech, now the diligent custodian of the Hannah Beswick story, wrote back to Baxter, explaining that there must have been an error in Mrs Gilbert Gorton's account, as Hannah Beswick's mother was a Robinson, not a Gorton, before her marriage. He enclosed a copy of the family tree provided by Edward Rhodes to help Baxter with his research. However, as there was a reference to someone with the name Gorton in Hannah Beswick's will – there is a bequest of a gown and a silver platter made to Ann, wife of Thomas Gorton, as well as £50 to Margaret, daughter of Thomas Gorton – he also sent a copy of the transcribed abstract.

Baxter wrote back in March 1949, effusively thanking Bosdin Leech and explaining that it was actually Hannah's *grandmother* who was a Gorton before her marriage. And, as he's sure Bosdin Leech will be very pleased to hear, 'the brocaded dress mentioned in the will was worn at a county ball as late as about 1860 by my cousin the late Mrs Gilbert Gorton'.[27]

No record of any further correspondence between Bosdin Leech and Stephen Baxter survives. I assume that, as I did when I first saw Baxter's letter, Bosdin Leech immediately checked the details of the bequest to Ann Gorton in Hannah Beswick's will. And I assume that he, like me, noted straightaway that the item in question was a 'brocaded silk *night*gown'. While it is (just about) conceivable that a woman went to a Victorian county ball dressed in a one-hundred-year-old nightdress, it does seem strange that Baxter didn't mention this very special connection to Hannah Beswick in his initial letter to R. U. Sayce, as Mrs Gilbert Gorton's visit to see the mummy in Manchester must have occurred around the same time as she was wearing the woman's nightgown to a party. It feels like that's something you would mention.

* * *

To return to 1890 and the Ghastly Find, the 'friend of a friend' element of the urban legend is well attested through continued recourse to the 'kinswoman of my mother' claims, from Mary Malin in 1877 to Mrs Gilbert Gorton in 1949. But to what extent can these versions of the story be described as an 'unselfconscious reflection of major concerns of individuals in the societies in which the legends circulate'?

In the immediate responses to the Ghastly Find, we see tantalizing details that evoke certain 'concerns' of the early 1890s. Superintendent Godby's evocation of 'the old "body snatching" days' and Dr Dearden's suggestion that Dr White 'purchased' a body for dissection might connect with the reappearance of body-snatching in popular culture. Robert Louis Stevenson's short story 'The Body Snatcher', which drew its inspiration from the story of surgeon Robert Knox and the criminals (such as Burke and Hare) who he employed to procure bodies for his anatomy lectures, was published six years before the Ghastly Find. The description of the mysterious coffin underneath the ancestral mansion might evoke vampire stories, pre-empting Bram Stoker's *Dracula* by just a few years. And when thinking about the murder of Patience Buckley – a woman with a name that seems tailor-made for horror fiction – by the butcher in Ashton-Under-Lyne, it's hard not to picture that butcher in a leather apron.[28] After all, the Jack the Ripper murders occurred two years before the Ghastly Find, and the ghoulish reporting of those crimes still dominated the popular press.

The circumstances of the Ghastly Find feel like the stuff of Victorian urban Gothic. In describing this particular mode of Gothic writing, Sara Wasson suggests that 'a dominant theme of urban Gothic is the incorrigible fragility of modernity: even triumphs of the built environment are precarious, and the collapse of edifices is often a metaphor for the psychological crumbling of those who dwell within them'.[29] And this seems an apt description for what is going on with the Ghastly Find reporting and response.

In June 1890, just a few weeks before the coffin was unearthed at Cheetwood, the *Manchester Weekly Times* had printed a story entitled 'A Curious Corner of Manchester'. The opening paragraph read:

> Of the thousands who daily pass along the two north roads out of Manchester it is safe to say that only a very small proportion have any sort of acquaintance with the little village built on the hill overlooking the Bury New Road, and spreading for some distance on the level land lying between the summit of this rising ground and Cheetham Hill Road. Cheetwood is a dreary place now, as are all survivals of scenes of rural beauty from which nearly everything that was either rural or beautiful has been taken away. Quite recently one of the old landmarks of this once pleasant outlying suburb of Manchester was demolished – Cheetwood Hall – the substantial front of which, a well-built house of the last century was seen from the Bury New Road. But this front was the screen of a much older and more interesting house, one which may have been built when a Tudor was King in England, for old records tell

> us that there was a Cheetwood manor in the reign of Henry VIII. Town extensions cannot, of course, but absorb the quaint old outskirts which tell of other times and other customs, but absorption generally means total destruction, and not, as in the case of Cheetwood, dismantlement and wreckage.[30]

Here we see a similar transition to that found in Hollinwood, where the once rural setting of Birchen Bower gave way to industrialization and urbanization, but with far more emphasis on the destruction and annihilation of the past.

Some history of Cheetham will help to explain the context for this somewhat brutal introduction to the 'wreckage' of Cheetwood.

In the Middle Ages and early modern period, Cheetham was a village and then a township to the north of Manchester. It was relatively large and prosperous, partly as a result of its proximity to the rivers, Irk and Irwell. The central 'district' of Cheetham became known as Cheetham Hill, and this area connected the township to neighbouring areas of Crumpsall and Broughton (rural areas that became well-to-do locations at the beginning of the industrial revolution, and the places where wealthy mill and factory owners would build houses to escape the smog and slums of Manchester). Around the edge of Cheetham were smaller villages, all of which had their own 'halls' (post-medieval manor houses built by the landed gentry): Strangeways, Cheetwood and Smedley. In 1485, Cheetham was granted to the Earl of Derby, and the earls continued to be the major landowners into the twentieth century.

However, a quick internet search or a conversation with a Mancunian will tell you that this is very far from how Cheetham is known today. The industrial revolution hit Cheetham like a ton of bricks and radically altered it.

Cheetham was one of the first townships to be incorporated into Manchester in 1838, when the larger town was granted its borough status. Again, this was partly to do with the prosperity of the township, and its usefulness as a link to Bury (via the Bury New Road, constructed by a turnpike trust in 1826) and the rest of Lancashire. Cheetham retained some level of independence for a time, with its own town hall being constructed in 1853 (the building survives but is now a restaurant), but eventually it became fully transformed into a suburb of Manchester.

What the area is perhaps best known for today, and the thing which shapes the character of modern Cheetham, is its cultural diversity. From the beginning of the nineteenth century, successive waves of immigration and settlement saw large Irish, Jewish, South Asian, Caribbean, Eastern European and – in more recent years – West and East African communities established in the area. Cheetham is now the home of Manchester Jewish Museum, various Eastern European social clubs, mosques, Catholic and Orthodox churches, Sikh temples, and possibly the most diverse retail offer in the city of Manchester.

In order for this transformation to occur, the old area had to be destroyed. Unlike with Hollinwood, this was not a gradual transition but rather, as the article from the *Manchester Weekly Times* suggested, an act of 'destruction'.

The areas around the Bury New Road were completely rebuilt, to the extent that it is no longer possible to identify older areas on a map. If you want to explain to someone now where Cheetwood once was, you have to say it was 'sort of' in the area between Derby Street and the Manchester Fort retail park. The only memory that survives is a single street name, Cheetwood Road, and a municipal park, Cheetham Park, which is a tiny (and unacknowledged) fragment of the old Cheetwood Hall grounds.[31]

What we see in the stories from 1890 is the immediate impact of this destruction. By this point, Strangeways Hall and its estate (a manor dating back to at least the fourteenth century) was completely gone, replaced by Strangeways Prison (now HMP Manchester), which was constructed in 1868 and designed by architect Alfred Waterhouse. Next to the prison was the earliest brickworks in the area, digging up the rich beds of clay underneath Cheetham to supply to expansive building projects in Manchester. Cheetham Hill Road (the Bury Old Road, or York Street as it was then called) had been constructed, with a series of new streets leading off from the left and right filled with houses.[32] Some older streets remained and were absorbed into the new town planning, although the evocatively named Dirty Lane was given the more respectable moniker of Elizabeth Street.

When Ordnance Survey mapped the area in 1888–89, the extent of the urbanization was clear, with tightly packed, grid-like residential streets stretching off from York Street and Elizabeth Street, before the area opened up again at its north end to the relative rural idylls of Smedley, Crumpsall and Broughton, a far cry from the large, impassive block marked out as 'Her Majesty's Prison' at the southern end. In between these areas, the Ordnance Survey map shows the last surviving bit of 'old' Cheetham – Cheetwood Hall and the remnants of its estate, with the incipient Derby Street cutting through the middle, and brick and metal works scattered around what was once fields and gardens.

In the 'Curious Corner of Manchester' report of June 1890, the *Manchester Weekly Times* notes that:

> The brickmakers have been laying siege to Cheetwood; for many years, they have been clearing and levelling the land, and now they are sapping the walls of the houses. Nay, some old homesteads that were once fair to see have completely disappeared, and the expanse of open land to the right, when the remaining houses are passed, is one vast melancholy field of broken clay.[33]

Any scholar of the Gothic would tell you that these circumstances are absolutely ripe for a return of the repressed, and so it's hardly a surprise to find, just one month later, a gruesome receptacle of human remains bursting out of the earth as the spectre of both the 'old body-snatching days' and the hall's former occupant.

There is something so much more brutal about the Ghastly Find story than the tone and style of the Birchen Bower legends, and I'd suggest this was the result of the ways in which the localities themselves changed. While Hollinwood managed to retain some of its older character, even with the imposition of factories, railways and mills, Cheetwood became a 'vast melancholy field of broken clay' before vanishing from the map completely. The site of the old hall is now hard to determine, but I think it was roughly on the site now occupied by Laherson Wholesalers, distributors of 'Stationery, Perfume, Health & Beauty, Batteries, Smoking, Electrical, DIY, Disposable, Baby Range, Pet, Household, Lighters, Seasonal, Pound Lines & More', on Sherbourne Street, a fitting monument to the 'incorrigible fragility of modernity'.

7
Ms Beswick

The coroner decided that he couldn't prove the lead box of 'tinned salmon' was human remains, by the way, so no further investigation was carried out. The remains were discreetly destroyed shortly after they were found, the brickworks continued, and the construction of Derby Street (started decades earlier and named after the landowner, the Earl of Derby) was completed. In 1860, brewer Joseph Holt bought a brewery site on the corner of Empire Street (formerly Exchange Street, which led up to the entrance of Cheetwood Hall until 1890), and, two years later, the Prestwich Poor Law Union built their offices next door to Cheetham Town Hall. In 1893, the Marks family moved to Cheetham Hill Road, and by 1901 Michael Marks (along with his new partner Thomas Spencer) had built a warehouse on Derby Street to serve their thriving new shop on Cheetham Hill. In 1910, after the England won the first ever European Ice Hockey Championships, the largest indoor skating rink in Britain – the Ice Palace – was opened across the road from the Marks and Spencer warehouse. The village of Cheetwood was gone, and the suburb of Cheetham Hill took its place.

After 1890, the significance of Cheetwood to the Hannah Beswick story fades. While the Ghastly Find story promised all sorts of Gothic gruesomeness, it's actually almost never mentioned in later retellings of the story. The ghost story of Birchen Bower remains a far more persistent image, perhaps because its location has remained in local memory, or perhaps because it has a less specific context than the Ghastly Find. Buried treasure and haunted barns are more broadly accessible concepts, and they require less background information than brick-works on land held in leasehold from the Earl of Derby in a part of the city that no longer exists.

Of course, Birchen Bower itself had also gone by the 1890s, but, as I've said, its name lingered in the name of the factory recreation ground ('The Bower'). Bower Lane continued to exist until the construction of the M60 motorway in the late 1980s, and a hotel nearby on Hollinwood Avenue was called The Bower Hotel until relatively recently (its name was changed to the Victoria Hotel, though it is still often known locally by its former name). People in Hollinwood and Failsworth still often recognize the location of Birchen Bower, even if it was better known as an electrical engineering plant for most of the twentieth century.

The memory of Miss Beswick's story also persisted through the twentieth century, mostly through retellings of (now) familiar versions of the story. For example, Edith Sitwell included a brief summary of the story of Miss Beswick in her book *English Eccentrics*, covering the mummification by Dr White, the taphophobia (romanticized as being terrified of falling into a 'a dreamless sleep'), and the large bequest to her embalmer, but adding in a description of Miss Beswick on her deathbed, 'with her white staring face, black menacing eyes, and thick black eyebrows'.[1] And the ghost story – following Dronsfield, Ingram and Frith – made a surprise reappearance in 1944 in *Good Morning*, a newspaper produced during the Second World War for the Royal Navy's submarine branch, which offered light-hearted stories, comic strips and 'pin-up girls' for the servicemen spending weeks under the ocean without contact with the outside world. The *Good Morning* version of the story pretty much reproduced the earlier accounts, including the buried treasure, Joe at Tamer's and the Satanic jubilee. It is notable only for the unexpected nature of the publication in which appeared and its idiosyncratic headline: 'She's a Tall Farmyard Phantom'.[2]

In 1966, a book by Harry Ludlam entitled *The Mummy of Birchen Bower and other True Ghosts* was published. The book's original cover appears to have been inspired by both Hammer Horror and the film posters for Universal's 1932 film *The Mummy*. An illustration depicts an old, apparently dead, and inexplicably green woman, swathed in bandages and propped up in a grandfather clock case, while a man in a purple velvet frock coat (looking not unlike Peter Cushing) gazes at her, clutching a white handkerchief in his hand.[3]

Nevertheless, the book's title story starts in a very different place than we might be expecting:

> The first report of strange happenings in the transformer department of the new Ferranti factory at Hollinwood, near Oldham, came from three men on weekend night shift who claimed to have seen a shadowy figure moving at one end of the shop. In April, 1956, when the hauntings at the factory were finally made public, there were no fewer than thirty-five night workers who claimed to have seen or heard the ghost.[4]

Ludlam goes on to explain that the ghost haunting Ferranti's was believed to be that of former resident Hannah Beswick, and he notes that the woman 'was believed to have haunted the spot for most of the two hundred years since her death'.

However, Ludlam seems reluctant to take the 'legend' at face value, and so he introduces an element not found in previous versions of the ghost story – research into the circumstances of the woman's life and death:

> The extraordinary story of Hannah Beswick, descendant of a very old Manchester family, is one of macabre human eccentricity combined with the eerily supernatural. It is also one which, by reason of the web of legends spun around it, developed over the years into a larger mystery baffling many investigators. Examination of these legends, together with reference to family papers and numerous other sources, enables us to construct a more accurate account of the affair, if some small mysteries still remain.[5]

Sadly, Ludlam's book doesn't have footnotes or references to the sources he has used, but his account of Hannah Beswick's life is strikingly more grounded in putative historical detail than previous accounts of the Legend of Birchen Bower.

Hannah Beswick (born in 1702) lived 'a comfortable life' at Birchen Bower with her half-brother John, who was two years younger than her. Their father had died in 1706, leaving his fortune to John. When her half-brother died in 1737, Hannah inherited his estate, including Birchen Bower, a smithy at Bradley Bent and a 'valuable freehold estate at Ashton-Under-Lyne'. By way of explanation, Ludlam clarifies that 'Birchen Bower was contained in the estate of Cheetwood-in-Cheetham'. He continues:

> In the years that followed Hannah seems to have lived a somewhat solitary existence at Birchen Bower, with its quaint four-gabled house built in the form of a cross. She never married, and it was probably by reason of her manorial status that she came to be popularly known as 'Madame Beswick'.[6]

What follows is a fairly faithful retelling of the 'legend' as set out by James Dronsfield in 1869, complete with the fear of the Pretender's army in 1745, the buried treasure and the request that her body not be buried. Ludlam supplements this with some biographical details about Dr White, including reference to Thomas de Quincey's memoirs. He also explains that Hannah's (half-)brother John had once almost been buried alive, and so Hannah had a 'morbid dread' of a similar fate.

When Ludlam moves on to discuss the afterlife of Hannah Beswick, both as a museum exhibit and as a ghost, he continues to ground his story in the 'real life' of its characters, using de Quincey's first-hand account of the mummy in the clock case at White's museum, for example. He covers the woman's alleged request to have her body periodically returned to Birchen Bower (resulting in paranormal phenomena in the granary), but again uses precise historic details to contextualize this:

> It is quite possible that Charles White, with his evident zeal for the curious, did transport the mummy to the estate on one or more occasions. If he took it there after the first twenty-one years, in 1779, it was during the lifetime of one or both of the executrices [of Hannah Beswick's will] with whom he was patently on familiar terms. If he took it there again after another twenty-one years, in 1800, it was during the ownership of the estate by three of his children; for in 1792, when the second of the executrices had died, Birchen Bower was leased to him by the Earl of Derby in favour of the children.[7]

He then goes through the now familiar accounts of hauntings at Birchen Bower, including the tall ghost who shot bolts of blue light from her eyes and the Satanic jubilee in the barn. He also notes that Hannah Beswick is buried in Harpurhey Cemetery – in grave 'number

223' – and that human remains were found 'under the floor of the drawing room in Cheetwood Old Hall' and were presumed to be 'those removed from her body when she was embalmed'. However, he then brings the story up to date:

> Today, with Birchen Bower vanished beneath modern factories and Hollinwood Avenue brightly lit with a steady stream of traffic, almost the only memory of the estate is perpetuated in the name of Bower Lane. All trace of Hannah Beswick and her ghost would seem to have disappeared. Unless, of course, the disturbances at the Ferranti factory in 1956 owe anything to her restlessness.[8]

In his careful combination of the 'Peter Street Mummy', the 'Legend of Birchen Bower', recourse to historic documents and knowledge of local geography (albeit with some minor inaccuracies), Harry Ludlam achieved what Robert Dukinfield Darbishire and E. Bosdin Leech had been unable to do: he wrote and published the true story of Hannah Beswick, the Manchester Mummy.

Case closed.

* * *

Or was it?

Ludlam's *The Mummy of Birchen Bower and Other True Ghosts* was republished as an omnibus edition with his 1967 book *The Restless Ghosts of Ladye Place and Other True Hauntings* in 1985. Just six years later, the World Wide Web was opened to the public, connecting the world with an information superhighway.

Given that a definitive account of Hannah Beswick's life and afterlife was published and available, and that the new 'universal linked information system' offered the potential for research beyond anything available to E. Bosdin Leech, let alone Robert Dukinfield Darbishire, you would be forgiven for assuming that the Manchester Mummy would enter the twenty-first century with a more defined identity. The internet would allow the story to be distributed more broadly, becoming something more than a Manchester curiosity or a Hollinwood legend, while also allowing the gathering of information and sharing of resources across more diffused platforms to resolve the 'small mysteries' that still remained.

It's fair to say that isn't what happened.

The twenty-first century hasn't quite known what to do with Miss Beswick. She doesn't really fit into academic discourse around museology, bioethics and cultures of death and dying, and popular retellings of her story have gone through so many replications and mutations that they are more jumbled than ever.

In recent years, serious academic scrutiny has been given to the practice of displaying human remains in museum collections, including the recent work by Angela Stienne on Egyptian mummies and the work of Simon Chaplin on the early history of medical museums.[9] Conversations (and arguments) are held – and openly – within both academic circles and the heritage sector about the appropriateness of displaying dead bodies in a museum setting, and about the possibility of further repatriation of unburied corpses. During the writing of this book, Routledge has published a new *Handbook of Museums, Heritage and Death*, with articles on historical context, curation practice, conservation issues, decolonization, 'shifting the perspective' and repatriation. Where the story of Miss Beswick appears in this discourse, it is as a footnote and, most often, with a repetition of an older account of the case (usually a version of de Quincey's or a citation of Jessie Dobson's 1953 article 'Some Eighteenth Century Experiments in Embalming', or both – which is strange, because Dobson's article refutes de Quincey's account quite conclusively).[10] However, it is mostly left out of the conversation completely.

The problem is that the story of Miss Beswick doesn't add enough to an academic enquiry to be worth following up. She wasn't removed from her grave by colonial treasure hunters, subjected to an 'unwrapping party' and separated from culturally and spiritually significant grave goods and funeral bandages. She wasn't forced to endure dehumanizing display in her lifetime, degraded in terms of both her race and her gender, before being commodified in death as an 'attraction'. Her body was displayed in a now-defunct public museum for a little over three decades, before being 'decently' buried in a municipal cemetery and left to rest in peace. Studies of early English experiments in embalming tend to focus on London and on the work of anatomists William and John Hunter, as there is far less material available on either provincial studies of medicine and anatomy (given that medical students prior to the nineteenth century had to go to London, Glasgow or Edinburgh in order to complete their training) or the careers of pioneering anatomists who had surnames other than Hunter. In this respect, Miss Beswick's embalmer is also a footnote, often appearing simply as a 'student of William Hunter' who went on to found a hospital in a provincial town and who died over fifteen years before the trial of Burke and Hare. Admittedly, Charles White does have a blue plaque in his honour on King Street in Manchester city centre, but this has little national, let alone global, interest.

In many ways, academic studies of heritage and death have treated Miss Beswick as she was treated during her time at the Natural History Museum – a local curiosity offering little beyond the incongruity of seeing a rich old woman from Manchester displayed next to the more intellectually and ethically challenging corpses of ancient Egyptians and decapitated Maori. It's a weird story, but there are many other cases that are more deserving of serious scholarly attention – such as the stories of Julia Pastrana and Saartje Baartman, which still have much to tell us about legacies of racism, slavery and colonization in the pursuit of scientific 'knowledge'.

The story of Miss Beswick is, therefore, relegated to the realm of the popular, rather than the academic, imagination. It's a weird story, and so it belongs alongside other weird stories, like the Highgate Vampire or Spring Heel'd Jack.[11] It's also a local story, and as such is better placed alongside tales of the Sad Cavalier at Middleton's Ring o' Bells pub or the screaming skull of Wardley Hall. Retellings of the story often end with recommendations for 'further reading', such as on the All That's Interesting website: 'After reading the spooky story of Hannah Beswick, the Manchester Mummy, read about the Japanese monks who mummified themselves while still alive. Then, learn about the Inca ice maiden, perhaps the most well-preserved mummy in human history.'[12] This really doesn't seem so far removed from George Head's enthusiastic account of visiting the King Street museum in 1834.

The internet offers rich opportunities for investigation and research, with thousands of archives, registers and documents now digitized and available (with or without a paywall). However, popular retellings of the Miss Beswick story are notable for their lack of new research. So, for example, we find web articles like 'Myths of Manchester: The Curious Tale of the Manchester Mummy', which opens:

> In 1688, Hannah Beswick was born in Cheetwood Old Hall to wealthy parents John and Patience. When her father died in 1706, she inherited his substantial wealth and moved to a stunning manor house in Hollinwood near Oldham called Birchen Bower.
>
> On the surface she lived a comfortable and privileged life but beneath the riches was a broken woman, traumatised by the unimaginable horrors that surrounded her brother John's 'death'.
>
> On the day of John's funeral, grievers were paying their last respects when a horrified spectator spotted something alarming. John's eyelid had flickered and upon examination by their family doctor, Charles White, he was declared alive.[13]

Or the entry for 'Manchester Mummy' on the Mummipedia Wiki, which states:

> Beswick's mummified body was initially kept at Ancoats Hall, the home of another Beswick family member, but it was soon moved to a room in Dr White's home in Sale, Cheshire, where it was stored in an old clock case. Following White's death in 1813, Beswick's body was bequeathed to a Dr Ollier, on whose death in 1828 it was donated to the Museum of the Manchester Natural History Society, where she became known as the Manchester Mummy, or the Mummy of Birchin Bower.[14]

The Manchester Mummy also has a Wikipedia page, which offers some overview of the 'facts', and offers a link to the page on 'Premature Burial' as background. It also (at the time of writing) cites Edith Sitwell's 1933 book as a description of the appearance and reception of the mummy at the museum and includes this paragraph:

> Hannah Beswick was born in 1688, the daughter of John and Patience Beswick, of Cheetwood Old Hall, Manchester. She inherited considerable wealth from her father who died in 1706. Some years before her own death, one of Hannah's brothers, John, had shown signs of life just as his coffin lid had been about to be closed. A mourner noticed that John's eyelids appeared to be flickering, and on examination the family physician, Dr Charles White, confirmed that he was still alive. John regained consciousness a few days later, and lived for many more years.[15]

The reference to John being Hannah's brother, and not her half-brother, and the suggestion of an additional sibling (though not named explicitly as Wright Beswick here) reveals either a reluctance on the part of the Wikipedia editors to include Ludlam's account of the case or a lack of awareness of its existence.

* * *

As mentioned in the previous chapter, stories about Miss Beswick were initially attached to specific locales for the purposes of creating a site-specific legend through which to cement the 'character' of an area (in the case of Hollinwood), bemoan the demise of a lost village (Cheetwood) or market an area to visitors (Sale). These tendencies resurface on occasions in the twenty-first century, despite the fact that Birchen Bower, Cheetwood Hall and Sale Priory are all long since destroyed.

In 2009, the BBC ran a short article on their website about the Manchester Mummy, which reads as a summary of other popular versions of the story, including the account of the brother who was revived after being placed in a coffin. The random date of the article – 11 August 2009 – isn't associated with any conceivable anniversary related to the story, which might suggest that the Manchester Mummy held such a place in the popular imagination that spontaneous retellings were inevitable. However, it's interesting to note the opening paragraph of the article: 'While Hollinwood's huge Hollywood-style sign may grab some fleeting attention, the area's first celebrity had fame that far out-lived her – for the most macabre of reasons.'[16] Sure enough, the website directs the reader to another article, published two hours earlier on 11 August 2009 and entitled 'Hollinwood Sign Apes LA's Rival', which reported on the appearance of an eight-foot high, sixty-foot long 'Hollinwood' sign made in the style of the iconic 'Hollywood' sign that appeared at the side of the M60 one day.[17] It is not inconceivable that, having reported on this quirky local news story about a little-known northern locale, a BBC writer was tasked with finding another curious tale of Hollinwood to accompany it.

One issue with this type of reporting, as with earlier retellings of the story, is that it can lack a firm grounding in local geography and history. The BBC sidesteps this issue by saying little about Hollinwood or the location of Birchen Bower, save for the implication that it is near Manchester and the link to a story that situates Hollinwood next to the M60 motorway.

Other accounts are less careful about evoking geographical or historical details, and these reveal another issue: a persistent amnesia about the history of the city of Manchester. This civic amnesia accounts for the lack of nuance in descriptions of Miss Beswick's fear of the Jacobite rebellion, for instance, as there is little collective memory about the complexities of the response to the arrival of Charles Edward Stuart's army in Manchester in 1745, and so we see it collapsed into the idea of widespread panic and even 'mass hysteria'.[18] All this denies the reality, where there was both hatred and support for the rebels within the town, with Bonnie Prince Charlie himself allegedly being put up in the house of Mr Dickenson on Market-sted-lane (now Market Street) for the duration of his stay. When the rebellion was quelled, and the Manchester men, such as Thomas Sydall and Thomas Deacon, who had supported the 'Pretender' were executed and their severed heads displayed on spikes in St Ann's Square, Dr Edward Hall (a colleague of Dr Charles White and a confirmed Jacobite) reportedly removed the heads one night and buried them in his garden.[19]

All this conflict and complexity is lost in a vision of a rich woman running scared of a 'foreign' army and burying her gold under the drawing-room floor. This myth persists because 1745 is so far outside living memory as to make anything possible.

The lack of memory or knowledge of the events of the '45 is perhaps understandable, given that almost nothing of mid-eighteenth-century Manchester now survives, and the Jacobite rebellion doesn't feature on school history syllabuses. However, there is another trend in reporting the Miss Beswick story that's just starting to emerge – a forgetfulness around the existence of the Natural History Museum.

The Peter Street museum led to the naming of the street at the side of the building. Museum Street is still there today, nestled between a building called St George's House and the dilapidated remains of the Theatre Royal. It's become something of a curiosity itself, appearing occasionally in local history articles about the background of certain street names. However, at times, the actual story of the museum that was on Museum Street becomes lost. For example, on the *Manchester's Finest* website, there is a brief explanation of the street name:

> A textile manufacturer in the 1800's called John Leigh Phillips was a collector of natural history artefacts. Following his death, the collection was taken by a group that would later become the Manchester Natural History Society in 1821.
>
> The society made their home in Peter Street in 1835 and showcased Phillips' assembly as an addition to a collection by the Manchester Geological Society. So, Museum Street now remains a tribute to Phillips and the society, despite there being no museum having been there at any point [*sic*].[20]

Even more dramatic is a story that appeared on the website *Movehut*, a site devoted to the commercial property market, in 2014. *Movehut* was reporting on the sale of St George's House, 'one of Manchester's most iconic buildings'. St George's House, as I've noted, sits on Peter Street next to Museum Street – it was built in the early twentieth century on the site of the former Natural History Society Museum. After getting the date of the Peterloo Massacre wrong, *Movehut* goes on to describe a strange incident in the history of St George's House:

> [D]uring the demolition of a previous building on the site, workers unearthed the mummified body of Hannah Beswick, better known as the Manchester Mummy. A wealthy woman with a pathological fear of premature burial, her body was embalmed after her 1758 death and kept above ground to be periodically checked for signs of life.
>
> Beswick's mummified body was eventually bequeathed to the museum of the Manchester Natural History Society, where she was put on display. In 1868 Beswick was finally buried in an unmarked grave at Harpurhey Cemetery – how her body came to be in the cellars of the Peter Street property remains a mystery.[21]

This description is almost comical in its misunderstanding, and there really is little danger at the present time of the Peter Street museum slipping out of memory entirely. The Manchester Museum – the museum of the University of Manchester – makes clear reference to both the museum and its location in material relating to its own history. Manchester's public library and archives service have illustrations of the Peter Street museum that circulate on websites and social media, as well as being used by more 'serious' press coverage, such as the BBC's story in 2009. However, the fact remains that the *Manchester's Finest* article and the *Movehut* story are still published versions of the Miss Beswick story. They may not be peer-reviewed or subject to any editorial intervention, but they have been added to the mix of versions of the story and are just as 'discoverable' as Harry Ludlam's more careful discussion of the case.

* * *

The Manchester Libraries image of the Peter Street museum serves as a reminder that the twenty-first-century internet is a very visual medium. A story rarely exists online without some accompanying images. The case of Miss Beswick poses a problem in this regard, as no images of the woman (in life or in death) exist. There are illustrations of the museum, as I've said, and also some sketches of Birchen Bower, Cheetwood Hall, Sale Priory and Dr White's house on King Street. Several images of Charles White survive, and these are sometimes (but definitely not always) included in versions of the Manchester Mummy story. In addition to this, web stories also include stock images of coffins, gold (for the buried treasure) and grandfather clocks.

At the time of writing, the Wikipedia page for 'Premature Burial' is illustrated with an image of Antoine Wiertz's 1854 painting 'The Premature Burial', which depicts a terrified-looking man pushing off the lid of a coffin in what appears to be a mausoleum and reaching out an arm. On the edge of the coffin are painted the words 'Mort du cholera. Certifié par nous Docteurs. Sansdoutes. [Died of cholera. Certified by us doctors. No doubts.]'. This picture is included on a number of web stories about Miss Beswick, acting as shorthand for 'fear of being buried alive'. For instance, 'Hannah Beswick, the Mummy in the Clock' on the *Historic UK* website, uses Wiertz's painting as its featured image (displayed above the headline), and also includes an illustration from an edition of Edgar Allan Poe's 'The Premature Burial', a painting of Charles White and a sketch of the Peter Street museum.[22]

Other (web)sites are somewhat more creative about how to represent a long-dead woman for whom we have no physical descriptions more reliable than 'thick black eyebrows' or 'tall farmyard phantom'.

While I have been working on this book, a new bar has opened in St George's House on Peter Street. The bar is called Exhibition, and it seems to be happy to be associated with the long-demolished museum and its notorious exhibit. In fact, the bar boasts a neon yellow installation depicting an almost classical-looking woman swathed in cloth, barefoot and possibly blindfolded, holding either a sack or a large hook in one outstretched hand. According to Exhibition's website, this is a depiction of Hannah Beswick, 'the local legend', as they 'like to think she watches over us today'.[23]

At the other end of the spectrum, a website entitled *The Ratbag Encyclopedia* – actually the blog and family history website of a man named Alan Thompson – has a post entitled 'Are You My Mummy?', which is mostly illustrated with images of maps, screenshots of digitized newspaper articles and images of Hollinwood as it is today. The article is a reasonably well-researched summary of different versions of the story, with the added element of Thompson's own family connection to Birchen Bower and a reference to Harry Ludlam's book. However, the featured image for the piece (which shows up as a thumbnail on internet searches) is a picture from Alfred Hitchcock's *Psycho*, showing the desiccated face of Norman Bates's mother superimposed onto the iconic shot of the Bates House.[24]

A further image that is currently circulating on the internet shows the face of an apparent preserved corpse, its teeth visible and the remains of some cloth or wrapping over its head, next to a grandfather clock (to the left) and a pile of gold coins (to the right). This image appears to originate with the article on the *Manchester's Finest* website, and it is an edited collage of two stock images with a picture taken from a *Ripley's Believe It or Not* article about a fake Egyptian mummy (made in Boston in 1923) in the Ripley's collection.[25]

When I began working on this book, the grotesque collage of a fake mummy with illustrative clock case and gold was where my summary of the ways in which Miss Beswick has been depicted was going to end. However, for a story that begins with 1830s travelogues, and takes in guidebooks, newspaper reports, pamphlets, ghost stories, professional correspondence, letters to the editor, websites and blogs, it seems right that the story of the Manchester Mummy has very recently made its leap onto another platform: TikTok. In a video entitled 'The Peculiar Afterlife of Ms Hannah Beswick', the account lifeandtimeshistory does an admirable job of condensing a summary of the case into the required short-form video format for the social media platform.[26] Narrating an overview of the case, including the taphophobia, the flickering eyelid of her brother John, the embalming by Charles White, storage in an attic (*not* on the roof) and eventual display in the museum, to the musical accompaniment of a Bach cello suite, lifeandtimeshistory ('James') appears in the bottom left-hand corner of the screen, while images and snippets of text appear in the centre to illustrate the story. The pictures are, by now, expected: a historic sketch of Harpurhey Cemetery, an illustration from Poe's 'The Premature Burial', Wiertz's painting, a movie poster for the 1962 adaptation of Poe's short story, a painting of Charles White, the blue plaque to Charles White on King Street, the sketch of White's King Street house, the sketch of the Peter Street museum, the 'Curious Interment' story from the *Manchester Guardian* in August 1868, a stock image of some mummified or desiccated hands. However, there is one further image, which appears at the beginning of the video and in the middle, which really captured my interest, as it was one I hadn't seen before.

The image shows what appears to be the dead body of an elderly woman, eyes closed and skin deeply wrinkled. She is wearing old-fashioned clothing, including a front-panelled embroidered dress with a white lace collar, and a cap with lace edging. The woman is bathed in an almost neon blue light. It is, I have to say, an intensely unsettling image, as the woman appears both lifelike and also unreal. The way her eyelids cover her eyes to reveal the shape of eyeballs underneath – unlike the images of either the Ripley's fake mummy or the Hitchcock film prop, which both have empty eye sockets – suggests the body of someone recently deceased or perhaps not even deceased at all. It wouldn't be hard to imagine one of those eyelids flickering.

An internet search revealed the source of the image, as it appears on a couple of other websites as well, and it brings us full circle. It's a photograph of a wax model of Miss Beswick in the Ripley's Believe It Or Not museum in Amsterdam. It is once again possible to visit Miss Beswick in a museum, albeit only to see a replica of the original mummy. And clearly wearing a dress, rather than the ticking that was reported at the time.

The information card on the display at the Amsterdam museum, written in Dutch and English reads:

> A TIMELESS LOVE STORY
> When Paula Beswick of Sale, England died in 1757, she left a fortune to her physician. To comply with her will, the doctor embalmed her body and kept it in a grandfather clock case where he could see it every day! Believe it or not!

I think the answer is: not.

As Jessie Dobson noted in 1953, the accounts that have been written about Miss Beswick, the so-called Manchester Mummy, are 'full of inaccuracies and contradictions'.[27] From implausible bequests (£25,000) that don't actually appear in her will, to fanciful tales of a brother (or was it a sister?) escaping premature burial due to the intervention of a doctor who, in truth, was only nine years old when John Beswick died for real, to buried treasure that was inexplicably never retrieved after the threat of Jacobite invasion receded, to an ever-shifting array of locations that are sometimes owned by Miss Beswick and sometimes by Charles White, to Mrs Gilbert Gorton's nightgown, a cedar tree brought from Lebanon, Mr Browne-Clayton's coffin and J. Wilfrid Jackson's work table, to a ghost that could shoot blue beams from its eyes, to Paula Beswick, Madame Beswick, Ms Beswick, and the spectres of Wright Beswick (the missing heir) and Patience Buckley (murdered by a butcher).

I'm not sure I believe any of it.

Part II

Life and death

8
Hannah

There is another place where we could start the story. We could begin here: with a girl born in Cheetham, Lancashire, at the end of the seventeenth century.

Hannah Beswick was born at Cheetwood Hall in 1694 to John and Hannah Beswick. She was baptized at the Collegiate Church (now Manchester Cathedral) on 10 February 1694, just six months after her parents' wedding in August the previous year. The couple married by licence, rather than banns, and it's quite likely that they knew their baby was on her way before they tied the knot.

Hannah's mother was Hannah Hadfield of Mottram-in-Longdendale, a village on the border between Cheshire and Derbyshire, and her maternal grandfather was Thomas Hadfield, who built Crowden Hall near the head of the Longdendale valley in 1692. Thomas died in 1697, leaving his infant granddaughter five shillings in his will – the first, but by no means the last (or the largest), inheritance Hannah would have in her lifetime.[1]

Tragically, Hannah's mother died when she was just one year old. Hannah Beswick (née Hadfield) was buried at the Collegiate Church on 7 November 1695. Her cause of death is not recorded, but given her age and the age of her first child – and the fact that no one else in the household died at the same time – I think it's very likely she died in childbirth or as a complication of pregnancy. Maternal mortality rates at this time have been estimated as high as 200 in every 10,000 births (meaning for every ninety-eight women who survived childbirth, two died), so this is a very plausible scenario. A common cause of maternal mortality was puerperal fever, or childbed fever, an infection of the uterus following childbirth. Sometimes known as the 'doctor's plague', puerperal fever was, sadly, commonly caused by doctors attending to an expectant mother, as a lack of understanding about germs and antisepsis meant that even simple hygiene measures such as handwashing were often not observed.

Whether Hannah Hadfield did give birth to a second child is unknown, as no record of a baptism survives and the child certainly didn't survive infancy. Hannah Beswick would remain an only child for some years to come.

Hannah's father was John Beswick, the son (and this will get confusing, I'm afraid) of John and Hannah Beswick of Cheetwood Hall. John's father (Hannah's paternal grandfather) died in 1685, leaving his widow to raise four 'dear and well-beloved' children who were all under the age of twenty-one, and so not old enough to inherit their father's property: John, Hannah, Francis and Esther.[2]

So, when Hannah was born, there were actually three (possibly four) Hannah Beswicks living together at Cheetwood Hall: grandmother, mother, child (and possibly aunt). Her father's youngest sister, Hannah's Aunt Esther, also lived at Cheetwood, and this was a relationship that would become a very important one for Hannah, particularly after the death of her mother.

Cheetwood was a hamlet on the southern side of Cheetham, a manor originally granted to the de Middleton family by King John (around 1212) but then held by the Cheetham and Pilkington families, before being granted to the Earl of Derby in 1485 and becoming recognized as a township. Cheetwood was bordered on its southern edge by Strangeways, the principal estate (aside from Cheetham itself) in the township, and both these hamlets had 'halls' by the fifteenth century – post-medieval manor houses leased by the landowner to members of the landed gentry or to yeoman farmers. In the late seventeenth century, when Hannah was born, Cheetwood and Strangeways – like most of the post-medieval manors in this part of Lancashire – were predominantly farmland, with grain crops (corn, wheat, barley and oats) giving way to cattle farming, which became the more lucrative use of arable land in pre-industrial South Lancashire.

Hannah's family leased Cheetwood Hall and its estate from the Earl of Derby. They lived in the manor house. There aren't any pictures surviving of the house from this time, but we can imagine what it might have looked like from both later accounts and comparison with other post-medieval manor houses in the area. It was likely a two-storey timbered building with gables, surrounded by 'gardens' (i.e. land planted and cultivated to shelter the house from the surrounding farmland, and to provide a kitchen garden to supply the family's domestic needs) and then pastureland, on which there would be a sprinkling of smaller cottages for the tenants who farmed the land.

But, for all its rural seclusion, Cheetwood at the turn of the eighteenth century was really a very well-connected place. It was incredibly close to the edge of Manchester, then itself a small town but one that was already rapidly developing. The Collegiate Church (a parish church with cathedral ambitions) and Chetham's Library (a public library founded in 1653 through a bequest by Humphrey Chetham, a wealthy merchant who was born at Crumpsall Hall, just a short distance from Cheetwood) were both only a short distance from Cheetwood.[3] Salford was a similarly short ride away to the west. And, depending on the whether or not the family approved of racing, Kersal (or Carsall) Moor was very close, offering the delights of the Whit Week Kersal Moor races on what is sometimes called Manchester's first racecourse, but is, of course, Salford's first racecourse.[4]

Cheetwood was close to the Bury road, the main route between Manchester and Bury at the time, going via Prestwich (where Hannah's uncle Francis would end up living after he married) and linking up with routes into Oldham.

Although no members of Hannah's family left a diary, other people living in the area in the first half of the eighteenth century did, and these allow a glimpse into the social lives of the upper middle classes at the time. Elizabeth Byrom (known as Beppy), daughter of John Byrom, was born in 1722 and kept a diary from August 1745 that was eventually found at Beppy's former home at Kersal Cell. Beppy Byrom's diary is mostly of interest now because its author was a Jacobite, a supporter of James II (deposed in the so-called Glorious Revolution of 1688) and his descendants' claim to the throne. Beppy was an enthusiastic supporter of Charles Edward Stuart, the grandson of James II who was also known Bonnie Prince Charlie or the Young Pretender, and her diary includes vivid descriptions of the arrival of the Pretender with his army in Manchester in 1745. However, her journal also gives an insight into social networks and entertainments of the time, with its very first entry noting a trip to Preston, followed by Blackpool 'for a ride by the sea-side'. Beppy's diary is an endless catalogue of movement, with family and friends travelling almost daily to 'drink tea', swap news or look after ill relatives.[5]

Perhaps a more mundane example is the diary of Dr Richard Kay of Walmersley, near Bury, the cousin of Samuel Kay, one of the founders of Manchester Infirmary. Richard Kay kept a diary from 1737 to 1750, and it's of interest now because that period includes his medical training at Guy's and St Thomas' hospitals in London, and Richard documented the lectures and teaching he received during this time. He also records his social life, and, like Beppy Byrom's diary, this is a near-constant series of visits, overnight stays, dinners and teas. For instance, he notes that one night he hosted a dinner party for Benjamin Gaskel and Peggy Hibbert from Manchester, Samuel Robinson and his sister Mary from Cheetham Hill, and his cousin Richard Kay from Chesham Lodge, with 'Musick and Dancing'.[6] Visits to and from Cheetham Hill appear regularly in Richard's diary, suggesting that it was not an unreasonable distance to travel for an afternoon tea or some dancing.

I don't know whether Hannah Beswick liked dancing. But I do know that when her mother moved to Cheetwood after she was married, she brought a virginal (a keyboard instrument similar to a harpsichord) with her. The instrument passed into Hannah's ownership on her father's death, being the second – not the largest, but possibly the most personal – inheritance Hannah would have during her life. Based on the surviving commonplace books of other seventeenth-century women, we might imagine Cheetwood Hall ringing with the sounds of hornpipes, sarabands and galliards.[7] I know other versions of Hannah Beswick's story have conjured the image of an ancient and eccentric spinster tending an isolated farm, but the image of a young woman playing 'Whoop, do me no harm, good man' on her mother's harpsichord at a house party is just as compelling.

Hannah's family got bigger in the years following her mother's death, as her father remarried. Hannah's stepmother was Patience Buckley of Grottonhead in Saddleworth. Patience was the daughter of John and Mary Buckley, and her family's wealth and class were very similar to that of Hannah Hadfield's family. It's quite possible that there was either a family relationship or a social connection between the Hadfields and the Buckleys. Both families were in John Beswick's social circle (given he married into both) and there are people with the surname Buckley mentioned in Thomas Hadfield's will. Mottram is just less than ten miles away from Saddleworth, on the Huddersfield road via Stalybridge. So it's plausible that Patience Buckley knew Hannah Hadfield before either of them became Mrs Beswick.

Patience Beswick (née Buckley) had one child with John Beswick, or at least one child that survived birth and infancy. Her son was named John, and he was Hannah's half-brother. But this family unit was sadly not destined to last long. In April 1706, when Hannah was twelve, her father died, leaving his estate in trust to his son John, who was only an infant at the time.[8] The executors of his will were his wife Patience and his sister Esther, who still lived at Cheetwood Hall with the family. Unlike Shakespeare, John Beswick left his best bed to his wife. His second-best bed went to his daughter Hannah, along with some furniture and the virginal that had belonged to her mother. John also ensured that the women in his family – his widow, daughter and unmarried sister – were financially secure, as even when his son reached the age of twenty-one and came into his inheritance in full, he was required to pay an annual payment to his female relatives for the rest of their lives.

One of John's executors, Hannah's Aunt Esther, would not stay at Cheetwood for long after his death. Esther Beswick married Joshua Robinson of Salford in November 1706, and their children Thomas and Mary would go on to have a close relationship with their cousins at Cheetwood.

John's other executor, Patience, would also not stay at Cheetwood. In 1713, when Hannah was nineteen and her brother was around ten, Patience Beswick (née Buckley) married John Shaw of Bradford. It's possible that Patience had gone home to her family after the death of her first husband, as her wedding to John Shaw was held at Saddleworth, not Cheetwood. Hannah's half-brother John would continue to have a strong connection to the Saddleworth and Oldham side of his family, making bequests to a number of his cousins on the Buckley side in his will and counting Robert Radclyffe of Foxdenton Hall in Chadderton among his friends.

It's not clear what Hannah did during this time. She may have gone to Grotton with her stepmother and half-brother, or she may have stayed at Cheetwood to be closer to her Aunt Esther. On reflection, the latter option is more likely, as Hannah's life as an adult would have much more connection to Manchester, Salford and the Robinson family, than it would to Saddleworth and Oldham or her maternal relatives in Mottram.

* * *

Hannah reached the age of twenty-one – 'full age' – in 1715. Hannah was born in England, but her adulthood was spent in the United Kingdom, the Act of Union being signed by England and Scotland in 1707 during the reign of Queen Anne. By the time Hannah entered adulthood, there was a Hanoverian king on the throne – George I – but there were also sustained attempts to remove the House of Hanover and restore the Jacobite monarchy. George I would go on to make a major decision that changed the political landscape of the country. He stopped attending meetings with government ministers, leaving decision-making powers in the hands of those ministers themselves. In 1721, this would lead to the recognition of a 'prime minister' (i.e. the one with ultimate power to run a government), with Sir Robert Walpole being the first man to hold this office.[9]

The country was facing financial, as well as political, transformation at this time. The South Sea Company had been founded in 1711 as public–private partnership intended to alleviate national debt through the trade and transportation of enslaved people from Africa to the 'South Seas' and South America. The dramatic rise and fall of the value of South Sea Company stock created an economic bubble that, when it burst, had a huge impact of the national economy. A parliamentary enquiry was held, revealing insider trading and bribery, and a number of rich politicians (to be fair, all politicians were rich in those days) were found to have profited personally from the creation of the bubble. The South Sea Company's crash (and, to an extent, its disgrace) led to its rival – a private company known as the Bank of England – becoming the banker to the British government.

Closer to home, Manchester was on the rise. In the 1720s, Daniel Defoe would describe the town as 'one of the greatest, if not really the greatest meer [mere] village in England', stating that, despite not having an MP or a corporation, this 'village' had a collegiate church, several parishes and a much larger population than you'd expect.[10] Manchester began the eighteenth century with a population of less than 8,000; it ended the century with a population of almost 80,000. Cotton would transform the greatest village in England into Cottonopolis, the world's first industrial metropolis, but this wouldn't happen during Hannah's lifetime. When Hannah was alive, fustian (cloth woven from cotton weft and linen warp) was king, with merchants (as Humphrey Chetham had done in the seventeenth century) becoming incredibly wealthy from the early textile industry and the associated property market.[11] Other fabrics – such as luxury silks, muslins and woollens – were produced and sold in such quantities in the eighteenth century that they became known (generically) as 'Manchester goods'.[12] Merchants capitalized on the boom in fabrics, but also diversified into other trades, including everything from wine to flower bulbs (in various attempts to rival the Dutch trade in tulips).

The religious landscape of Manchester was also changing. A 'Dissenters' Meeting House' had been founded in Manchester in 1694, the year Hannah was born. This chapel, probably the first building erected for non-conformist worship in Lancashire, was constructed on a site called Plungeon's Meadow in what is now Manchester city centre. A non-conformist congregation was founded in Manchester by Rev. Henry Newcome, a Presbyterian preacher at the Collegiate Church who was expelled from his living on 'Black Bartholemew's Day' 1662 because of his refusal to give 'unfeigned assent and consent' to the Book of Common Prayer and the Thirty-Nine Articles. Newcome's congregation worshipped for a time in a barn on Shudehill, but, when funds were raised, Plungeon's Meadow was bought for the purpose of constructing a new meeting house, known as the Cross Street Chapel.[13]

Religion, politics, economics and monarchy were closely intertwined. The Collegiate Church was perceived to have High Tory and Jacobite sympathies, whereas the non-conformist congregation was generally supportive of the Hanoverian succession. A gang of Jacobites led by a man called Sir John Bland attacked the Dissenters' barn on Shudehill in 1687, smashing the windows and disrupting the service. How frustrating it must have been for Sir John when, only a few years later, his wife Ann (along with her parents Sir Edward and Dame Meriel Mosley) became one of the most generous contributors to the new chapel. Ann Bland was the heiress to the Manor of Manchester, and, after the death of Henry Newcome, she founded a new parish church for Manchester. Work on the church began in 1709, and in 1712 Manchester's new church was consecrated as St Ann's – partly dedicated to St Anne, the mother of Mary, and partly as a tribute to its founder, Lady Ann Bland. In the 1720s, the area around the church was planted and designed to resemble squares in the fashionable towns of London and Bath, and it became known, obviously, as St Ann's Square.

The establishment of St Ann's Church and St Ann's Square, and their popularity with the fashionable elite of the town, led to further developments in the surrounding area, with the first exchange being built close by (near the site of the surviving Royal Exchange, which is now a theatre rather than a trading floor) and James's Square, another fashionable square built just behind St Ann's Church (and allegedly named for the Jacobite cause, in response to the perceived Hanoverian bias of St Ann's), becoming *the* hot property of the 1730s and 1740s.[14]

It's hard to say whether Hannah Beswick was especially aware of any of the political or religious conflicts going on in Manchester and across the country at the beginning of the eighteenth century. Was she aware of the coronation of Queen Anne when she was eight years old? Or that when the Queen regnant died the line of succession was a source of conflict and dispute? She is more likely to have been aware of the coronation of George I (when she was twenty), but did she know that it was accompanied by rioting in various towns across England?

Was Hannah a supporter of the Hanover succession, like Lady Ann Bland? Or was she a Jacobite, like Beppy Byrom?

Perhaps she didn't care. Perhaps this political and religious unrest didn't touch her day-to-day life in the slightest. But she certainly chose to indulge in some of the tangential benefits of all this upheaval and change – Hannah bought herself a nice house on King Street.

* * *

But I'm getting ahead of myself. Hannah obviously didn't buy a townhouse with her father's second-best bed. In order to understand her move into the fashionable property market of 'the greatest village in England', we have to go back a couple of generations.

Hannah's paternal grandfather, John Beswick, was a gentleman. By that I mean, he was a member of the lowest echelon of the gentry. On the other hand, Hannah's maternal grandfather, Thomas Hadfield, was a yeoman, the class just below gentry but above husbandman. A full understanding of the nuances of this difference requires a complex analysis of the history and development of the English class system from 1066 onwards, and there simply isn't room for that here. I'm going to simplify things here and just focus on the aspect of the class system that matters most to Hannah's story: ownership of land.

In a nutshell, to be a 'gentleman' (which meant you didn't work for a living and, from 1430, you had the right to vote), you had to own land *freehold* that brought in more than 40 shillings a year in rent. A 'yeoman', while possibly just as wealthy (if not wealthier) than a 'gentleman', had land in *leasehold* from either the lord of the manor or a gentleman freeholder. Neither gentlemen nor yeoman had hereditary titles or peerages, though many would aspire to (or acquire) knighthoods or baronetcies in their lifetimes that would confer hereditary status on their descendants. And both gentlemen and yeoman could rent out their land to subtenants, potentially bringing in sizeable income in rents.

As I've said, Hannah's family had Cheetwood Hall and its demesne (the land attached to the manor and retained for the owner's use) in leasehold from the Earl of Derby, making her grandfather a leaseholder, not a freeholder, in Cheetham. However, he also owned the freehold on other estates in Lancashire, including Birchen Bower, Claytons and Bradley Bent in Hollinwood and an estate in Ashton-Under-Lyne. These were the 'country estates' of the Beswick family, which conferred the status of gentleman upon their owner, even if he lived in a manor house on leasehold land elsewhere in the county.

Thomas Hadfield, on the other hand, was a leaseholder of the land on which he would build Crowden Hall and, therefore, a yeoman. Similarly, Hannah's stepmother's family, the Buckleys of Grottonhead, were tenants of the freeholder and therefore yeomen. However, by 1716, the family had acquired freehold land at Saddleworth, allowing at least some of them to style themselves as gentlemen. The Buckleys are a good example of a family on the border of class categories, as they seem to switch between yeoman and gentleman between generations. When Patience Buckley's mother Mary (the maternal grandmother of Hannah's brother John) died in 1724, she described herself as a yeoman in her will.

The fact is, though, that John Beswick, Thomas Hadfield and Mary Buckley were all really rich, rich enough to make the issue of freehold versus leasehold seem like a triviality. Forget about the land for a moment, these families were cash rich. And I mean that quite literally. When John Beswick (Hannah's grandfather) died in 1685, an inventory of his property revealed that he had £16 in gold in his house, £60 'in one bagg att home' and £210 'in another bagg att home'. That's the equivalent of around £35,000 today, in cash, in a bag in his house.

John Beswick, like the Hadfields and the Buckleys, used this money to buy more property. For instance, shortly before his death, he purchased the old manorial bakehouse, a building that had once been the 'common oven' of the town of Manchester, which had belonged to the lord of the manor who would charge his tenants a fee to come and have their bread baked. By 1684, when John Beswick purchased it, the oven was no longer a common bakehouse but had been converted into a dwelling-house and land that was tenanted by a Miss Francis Frickland. John Beswick was now Miss Frickland's landlord and would collect a rent from her.[15]

When John Beswick died, neither of his sons were old enough to inherit his estate, and so he left it in trust to his widow (Hannah's grandmother). As a widow, Hannah could exercise financial control of the estate, managing it on behalf of her oldest son until he came of age. So, in 1698, Hannah sold the old bakehouse on to Manchester Grammar School, who converted into a house for the High Master. I like to think that she made a profit on the deal.

Hannah's grandmother died intestate in 1702, but as her eldest son (Hannah's father) was now 'of age', the estate that had belonged to his father passed to him in its entirety. Hannah's grandfather had made financial provision for his younger children – her aunts Hannah and Esther and her uncle Francis – but the estate was always intended to pass to his first-born son. In turn, Hannah's father bequeathed the estate to his first-born son, despite the fact that his daughter was older. This was the first – not the last, but definitely the largest – inheritance Hannah's brother would have in his lifetime.

I say not the last, because John (Hannah's brother) also inherited land from his stepfather. Patience Shaw (née Buckley, formerly Beswick) died in November 1717, and her husband John Shaw died the following month. The couple had no children together, so John Shaw left his property to his stepson and his brother-in-law (the husband of his wife's sister). On the death of his stepfather, John Beswick inherited land in Yorkshire.

One final word on land tenure as relates to John Beswick's inheritance. The Cheetwood property was leasehold, and the Chadderton properties were freehold, but other properties were held by the family in copyhold. Copyhold was an archaic form of leasehold, harking back to the feudal system. Originally, copyhold lands were occupied by 'villeins', non-freemen who were bound in service to the lord of the manor. Villeins could occupy a portion of land and cultivate it for their own use, but only at the pleasure of the lord of the manor. This became codified as a form of land tenure, with transfer of the right to occupy the land being added to court rolls and a copy being made for the tenant as proof of their rights. By the seventeenth century, there were no villeins, and copyhold lands were now often held by gentlemen or yeomen, possibly after generations of social mobility had transformed the status of the tenant, but not the status of the tenure. Copyhold became a sort of ceremonial version of leasehold, in which, when a copyholder died, their heir had to present themselves at the manorial court, hand the rights of the land back to the lord and request that it be transferred to them. Due to its history, copyhold did retain its requirement that a tenant act in servitude to the lord, but by the end of the seventeenth century this was more a token gesture than bonded labour.

And so, by 1717, Hannah's brother John had inherited quite a complex property portfolio, including freehold estates, a leased manor house and copyhold lands in Yorkshire and Derbyshire. All of this was held in trust until he was twenty-one, by which time he had also inherited ten pounds from his grandmother, Mary Buckley.

* * *

By the 1730s, Hannah's brother was living at Birchen Bower, an estate in Hollinwood, Chadderton. If – and it's only an *if* – we are to believe stories about an old barn on the estate with a timber beam inscribed 'I.B. 1728', then we can assume that stands for John Beswick.

Hannah didn't live with her brother at Birchen Bower. In fact, there's only a little circumstantial evidence that she ever lived there.

By 1737, John Beswick lived at Birchen Bower with his cousin Mary Robinson (who would have been in her twenties at this point). Mary was the daughter of Hannah and John's Aunt Esther, their father's younger sister who had lived with them at Cheetwood when they were children. It's not clear why Mary lived with her cousin, but I assume that as a single man in possession of a good fortune, John Beswick was in want of a housekeeper. It's interesting that his unmarried sister didn't perform this role for him, but perhaps Hannah had better things to do.

John Beswick died in 1737, unmarried and without children. The property portfolio he had inherited from his father and stepfather had to be bequeathed to an appropriate heir and, with the exception of some small portions of property that passed to male relatives on his mother's side, John willed the whole lot to his sister.

The will of John Beswick is one of the first clear indicators that we have to Hannah Beswick's character. John clearly believed that Hannah should not only inherit his estate, but also that she would know how to manage it. He left instructions about bequests to relatives who were not yet twenty-one, stating simply that his sister would be able to deal with these when the time came. He did make smaller bequests to male relatives – Thomas Robinson, Mary's brother, on his father's side, and various Buckleys and Saxons on his mother's – but the vast majority of his estate was willed outright to his older sister and, significantly, he stated clearly that it was his intention that his sister be entirely free to bequeath the lands in turn *however she wanted*.

John Beswick's executors were his sister, his cousin John Saxon of Audenshaw (the son of his mother's sister and a yeoman) and his friend and neighbour Robert Radclyffe of Foxdenton Hall (an esquire, one up from a gentleman). Interestingly, both of the men immediately relinquished their executor roles after John's death. No reason for this decision is given on the court documents, but on 1 May 1738, Robert Radclyffe and John Saxon stepped back and gave complete administrative control of the estate to Hannah Beswick.

This was the largest inheritance Hannah would have during her lifetime.

Now, various accounts of Hannah Beswick's story will tell you that, at this point in her life she entered into a reclusive and solitary life at Birchen Bower, farming the land, burying treasure under the floorboards, and being frightened of both Bonnie Prince Charlie's army and being buried alive. What actually happened was that she bought a house on the most fashionable street in Manchester.

I'm not going to try and make the claim that Hannah was some sort of fashionista or socialite. Her wardrobe when she died included the sort of nice clothes a woman of her class might own – some Brussels lace, a tabby gown, a grey silk negligée – and, while a claim has been made that she was 'fashionable' in her apparent enjoyment of tea (evidenced by her collection of thirteen silver teaspoons and tea tongs), this is probably stretching the point.[16] Tea drinking had been popular with the upper classes since the 1680s, and surviving diaries from Hannah's contemporaries make it clear that 'drinking tea' was a fairly standard part of any social visit. Admittedly, tea imports to England quadrupled during Hannah's lifetime, but it's difficult to view the woman as cutting-edge just because she owned some teaspoons.

What the thirteen teaspoons – along with the other silver plate at Hannah's house, and her mahogany carding table and oak dining set – shows more clearly is that she did some entertaining at Cheetwood. This is the paraphernalia we would expect of a normal well-to-do eighteenth-century life, I think, not the hoarded treasures of an eccentric. There is almost a mundanity to Hannah's (undoubtedly comfortable) life, with its silverware, feather beds and silk brocaded nightgowns. I'll admit that when I first read Hannah's will and the inventory of her possessions, hoping for a glimpse of the woman who would become a 'legend', I was disappointed. What I saw, on first reading, was a rich spinster who passed her time drinking tea and playing cards with her relatives. An unremarkable life, as so many people have claimed.

The thing is though, rich unremarkable spinsters from eighteenth-century villages near Manchester don't generally end up as museum exhibits.

9
Sundry odd things

When Hannah Beswick died at the age of sixty-four, she left a long and detailed will. As an unmarried woman, with no children but with a large property portfolio, she had to ensure she left clear and unequivocal instructions to ensure inheritance.

Hannah Beswick's will has been of interest to later generations for two reasons. The first is that there have been claims that she either left instructions about keeping her body above ground after death, or a substantial bequest to Dr Charles White. The second reason is that there have been suggestions that the ownership of Birchen Bower is somehow contested or ambiguous. Anyone reading Hannah's will for proof of these claims will be sorely disappointed.

Hannah's will left the administration of her estate to three executors: Charles White, Mary Greame and Esther Robinson. A fourth person, John Whittaker, is named, not as an executor but as someone entrusted with ensuring that certain legacies were paid or effected. The leasehold lands at Cheetwood were left to Mary Greame, for the duration of her natural life, and then to Charles White and his heirs in perpetuity. Lands in Chapel-en-le-Frith in Derbyshire were left to her cousin on her mother's side, John Hadfield, and copyhold lands in Yorkshire inherited from her brother's stepfather were left to Edmund Beswick of Blackley (a cousin on her father's side) and his wife Ann, for use during their lifetimes, and then to Ann Ogden, the granddaughter of her uncle Francis, and her heirs. Birchen Bower, Bradley Bent, Claytons and some land in Droylsden were left under a complicated set of instructions to the descendants of Hannah's cousin Thomas

Robinson (son of her aunt Esther), under which the lands were to be held in trust by John Whittaker and Charles White. The trustees were instructed to pay the income from the land to Thomas Robinson, and then to maintain his children until the youngest was twenty-one, at which point the Droylsden property would pass into the ownership of Thomas's oldest son, John (and his heirs forever), and Birchen Bower, Bradley Bent and Claytons into the possession of Thomas's second son, Thomas the younger, for his remainder of his life. After Thomas the younger died, the estates would go to his first-born son, but if this son died before he reached twenty-one, it would go to his second-born son, and so on through all of his hypothetical sons and then all of his hypothetical daughters. If Thomas the younger had no children who reached the age of twenty-one, then the income from the estates would go to the first-born son of Thomas Robinson's third son, Peter Robinson, for the remainder of his natural life, and then to his first-born son, but if this son died before he reached twenty-one ... etc., etc. Hannah's will then continued in this vein through all the children of her cousin Thomas Robinson – John, Thomas, Peter, Joshua, Esther and Ann – and all their hypothetical offspring, leaving you with the feeling that this freehold is not so very free at all. However, the reason for this long and drawn-out document was clearly to ensure that daughters weren't disinherited if no sons were born.

The will was challenged by Hannah's cousin Thomas (the elder), in a lawsuit pursued in 1761 and then another in 1774, but this seems to have had little to do with the entail on the properties. As well as property bequests, Hannah left several other legacies to her cousin's children, including monetary payments and financial support for apprenticing the boys to appropriate professions. Joshua, Thomas's youngest son, died in infancy shortly after Hannah's will was proved, and his father pursued lawsuits to get a share of Joshua's intended financial inheritance as his 'lawful next of kin'.

While all this goes some way to refute the stories that circulated in the nineteenth and twentieth centuries about Hannah's will, it's not actually very interesting. Birchen Bower would, in the end, be inherited by the son of Thomas Robinson the younger, Joshua Kay Robinson. This Joshua died in 1828, by which point two of his sons had moved to Delaware in the United States and his eldest daughter had moved to the Isle of Man. In 1834, Joshua's widow, Ann Robinson (née Whitehead), cut Birchen Bower up into portions and sold them off to the highest bidder. The description in the auction information said:

> The above property is situated on each side of Bower Lane, and a great portion thereof is contiguous to the village of Hollinwood, and lies very near to the turnpike road leading from Manchester to Oldham, and presents several most eligible sites for building factories or dwelling-houses, being in the midst of a manufacturing district, and distant about three miles from Oldham and four from Manchester.[1]

Ann Robinson clearly struggled to sell of the entire property, as she still had nine acres of it left in 1839. This last bit of Birchen Bower was offered up for as a rental property by its owner, a woman who was, according to the advertisement she placed in the newspaper, 'declining the farming business'.[2] Nevertheless, some memory of Hannah Beswick remained at Birchen Bower – not a headless ghost or a tall farmyard phantom, but the fact that the last of Thomas Robinson's descendants to live at Birchen Bower, Joshua Kay Robinson, named his eldest daughter Hannah Beswick Robinson.[3]

* * *

If you're looking for someone with a secret treasure hoard hidden from her relatives, or someone scared of being buried alive, Hannah's will is not the place to look. The vast majority of it is taken up with mind-numbing legalese about the succession of Birchen Bower, Claytons and Bradley Bent.

However, if you're looking for indications that Hannah Beswick was something other than your average tea-drinking spinster, it makes for rather charming reading.

Firstly, Hannah's choice of executors is somewhat idiosyncratic. She names three people: Charles White, Mary Greame and Esther Robinson, plus John Whittaker who is to act in an administrative role, holding the trust for the freehold lands along with Charles White, and ensuring that her cousin's sons are apprenticed to appropriate trades.

Two of these people are easy to explain. John Whittaker was the widower of Hannah's cousin Mary. Mary Robinson, the sister of Thomas

Robinson who lived with John Beswick at Birchen Bower until 1737, married John Whittaker, yeoman of Strangeways, in 1747. The couple didn't have any children, and Mary died before 1758. Esther Robinson was the eldest daughter of Hannah's cousin Thomas, and therefore niece to John Whittaker. Given that a large amount of Hannah's estate (both cash and property) was going to the family of her cousin Thomas, it's not so strange to find the man's brother-in-law and daughter acting as executors. And yes, some may question why Hannah chose Esther, and not John, Thomas's eldest son, but it's not the weirdest thing about the will.

Charles White and Mary Greame, on the other hand, aren't related to Hannah. The people to whom Hannah bequeathed Cheetwood Hall, as well as some sums of money and personal effects, weren't members of her close family.

The received version of the story is that Charles White was Hannah's family physician, who tended to her so well during an illness (and possibly also saved her brother John from a premature burial) that she rewarded him with a lavish gift in her will. It certainly seems that the doctor *did* tend to Hannah during an illness, as a payment of £10 10s for 'attending to the testatrix in her illness' was made from her estate after death. She also left him a cash bequest of £100, and the lease of Cheetwood Hall after the death of Mary Greame. However, Charles White is unlikely to have been Hannah's *family* physician, as he was only born in 1728 and so could not have tended to her parents or her brother. So how did Hannah come to know the good doctor?

I have two theories. The first is that Charles White was known to the Robinson family. Samuel Kay, one of the founders of the Manchester Infirmary along with Charles White, lodged with a Thomas Robinson of Salford for a time while he was completing his medical training. It's possible that this Thomas Robinson was Hannah's cousin, and that Samuel Kay was known to the Robinson family.[4] If Samuel Kay knew the Robinsons, then, perhaps, the family introduced Kay and White to their wealthy cousin Hannah. I'll return to this theory later on.

The second theory brings us back to that house on King Street. In her will, Hannah left a house on King Street, Manchester, to Esther Robinson and then to John Robinson (Esther's brother) after her death.

Hannah did not inherit this house on King Street in her brother's will, so she must've bought it after his death.

As I've said, James's Square, later King Street, started to become a very desirable street after the construction of St Ann's Church and St Ann's Square. Its first residents were wealthy and influential people of the town, including Dr Peter Mainwaring, one of the first physicians at the Manchester Infirmary, who had a townhouse built on the square in 1736.[5] Peter Mainwaring was good friends with John Byrom, though the two men disagreed about the monarchy. Mainwaring was a Hanoverian, whereas Byrom, as I've said, was a Jacobite. In the '45, Jacobite rebels broke into Mainwaring's house on King Street, which even Beppy Byrom (despite being an enthusiastic supporter of the Pretender's army) thought was 'a little rough'.[6]

Also living on King Street in the mid-eighteenth century were Richard Hall, a student of anatomist William Hunter and one of the original members of the Manchester Literary and Philosophical Society, who would go on to found Manchester's Lying-In Hospital with Charles White in 1790. Richard's brother Edward Hall was the man who supposedly removed the spiked heads of Thomas Sydall and Thomas Deacon from St Ann's Square in order to give them a decent burial. And there was also Thomas White, midwife, surgeon and father of Charles White. Thomas White lived with his family – his wife Rosamund, daughter Sarah and son Charles – at a house on the corner of King Street and Cross Street that had been built by a Mr George Croxton. Thomas practised medicine from the King Street townhouse until his retirement to Sale Priory, when his son took over the Manchester practice.

Given that we know Hannah bought a house on King Street at some point between 1737 and 1757, Thomas White – and later his son Charles – would have been her neighbour. Was it perhaps Hannah who introduced her cousin Thomas to Samuel Kay, rather than it being the other way around?

Hannah is unlikely to have bought a house on King Street just to be close to the prominent medical men of the town. It's much more likely that she was attracted by the desirability of the street and its proximity to the most fashionable areas of the town. For instance, in 1744–45, Manchester's first ever public concert series took place in town, and a number of the King Street and St Ann's Square residents were in attendance. A series of sixteen subscription-funded concerts were held, featuring music by Corelli, Tessarini, Vivaldi and other baroque composers. Hannah wasn't on the list of subscribers for the first concert, though some of the names we've seen already were, including Robert Radclyffe of Foxdenton, Mr and Mrs White, Dr Mainwaring and a Mr Robinson, who subscribed for two people (frustratingly without a first name, so I can't say if this was one of our Robinsons, or who his guest was). After the fourth concert in the series, the subscription system was altered, and tickets appear to have been sold around the town without a record being kept of all the attendees.[7]

There's no getting away from the Jacobite rebellion, as promotion of these concerts was largely led by supporters of the Jacobite cause. The name '*Mr Anonymous*' appears on the list of subscribers, and it has been suggested that this was none other than Bonnie Prince Charlie himself: 'Can the *Mr Anonymous*, whose name appears in the above list of subscribers, have been Prince Edward, who might thus *incognito* join the Manchester gentry in the enjoyment of these new and, to them, delightful entertainments?'[8]

However, the concerts themselves don't seem to have been particularly partisan. On the list of subscribers for the first event is Dr Mainwaring, the staunch Hanoverian whose house was invaded by Jacobites after he urged the men of Manchester to arm themselves against the rebellion. But we also find the Byroms and the Halls, families firmly in the Jacobite camp, on the list, suggesting that Manchester's two teams were happy to come together for a society occasion. At least, they were until June 1745, when the number of attendees for the concerts dropped dramatically. Writing a century after the event, John Harland suggested that 'the rebellion had begun to array the whigs [Hanoverians] and the jacobites against each other, so that they could not meet, even in public, on friendly terms'.[9]

Assuming we've dropped the idea of buried treasure at Birchen Bower now, there is still a question around how Hannah responded to the '45. I would suggest three possible narratives for what Hannah was doing at this time. The first is that she – whether a Hanoverian or a Jacobite – was indeed living at King Street during 1745, in the thick of the action, waving on the Pretender's army (like Beppy Byrom) or condemning them (like Sir John Bland and Dr Mainwaring). Perhaps she, like many of the residents of King Street, continued to enjoy the social life of the town, even in the midst of the rebellion, and perhaps she even attended one of the 'new and, to them, delightful entertainments'.

The second narrative is that Hannah did indeed retreat to Birchen Bower to avoid the impending arrival of the Jacobites. I don't mean that she was gripped by 'mortal dread', but rather that the inconvenience, disruption and potential for violence was just not something she wanted to see. She wouldn't have been the only person to make the decision to head out to a country estate to avoid chaos in town. For instance, Samuel Kay, a Hanoverian, left Manchester for his family's estate in Bury.[10] In his assessment of Kay's decision, E. M. Brockbank suggests that anyone, whether Hanoverian or Jacobite, 'who could manage it, left the town to avoid the rebels'.[11] Is that what Hannah did in 1745?

Although, by Hannah's death, Birchen Bower was rented out to two tenants, there is some evidence that Hannah spent time there during her lifetime. In the inventory produced for Thomas Robinson's challenge to the will, most of Hannah's possessions, including personal items like family pictures, dressing tables and a looking glass, are listed as being in Cheetwood Hall. However, there are some 'sundry goods' listed at Birchen Bower, including bedding, an oak chest, a pewter tankard, an easy chair and thirty bottles. There's quite a distinct difference between these 'sundry goods', and the more practical and sociable arrangements of Cheetwood Hall, but it's still conceivable that the items are remnants of a previous stay at the house.

The third narrative is that Hannah never went anywhere. The house on King Street was an investment, not her home, and so it was rented out to a tenant. Hannah didn't go to town, but she didn't go to Birchen Bower either. The events of 1745 were not even on her radar. She stayed at Cheetwood Hall, drinking tea and playing cards with her cousin Mary Robinson. Or, perhaps, with someone else called Mary.

* * *

The other executor of Hannah's will, Mary Greame, has generally been overlooked in discussions of the Hannah Beswick story. On the whole, people have lumped her in with Esther Robinson, assuming that she was a young member of Hannah's family – sometimes erroneously described as 'her mother's relations', as we've seen.

When I first saw Hannah's will, I also assumed this. I found it surprising that Hannah made two young, unmarried women executors of her will. I thought that this was maybe an example of what Jolene Zigarovich has described as 'matriarchal economies' that 'emerged in [eighteenth-century] wills in which women wielded their power by directing their own inheritances to deserving daughters and female relatives'.[12] Zigarovich expands on these 'matriarchal economies':

> Bequests given by women to daughters, granddaughters, nieces, and female servants and friends indicate not only the increasing importance of self-fashioning in the process of writing or dictating a will and choosing items (however small) to bequeath, they also reveal how the female testator can bestow economic power on other women.[13]

In this light, it's interesting to revisit the lengthy entail on Birchen Bower. It appears that this was written to ensure that daughters weren't automatically disinherited because of their sex. If the heir to Birchen Bower didn't have any sons, the estate would pass to his (or her) eldest daughter *and her heirs*, not to the nearest male relative.

In her will, Hannah left a lifetime tenancy of her house on King Street to Esther Robinson, and a lifetime tenancy of Cheetwood Hall to Mary Greame. Esther was also in the line of succession to Birchen Bower, as the eldest daughter of Thomas Robinson. Hannah also made a series of personal bequests to her executors, including a brown silk negligée and petticoat to Mary, and a picture of 'her grandmother' (Hannah's Aunt Esther) to Esther. There were also a number of other bequests to women and some fairly specific instructions for Mary, Esther and another woman called Sarah Jenkinson, which I'll come to shortly.

Hannah had no children, but she also had no nieces and nephews, as her only brother also died childless. It makes sense that she would choose to bequeath her considerable fortune to the children of her cousin Thomas, as these were the nearest relatives she had. It's also testament to the relationship that Hannah and John enjoyed with their Robinson relations.

However, Mary Greame wasn't one of these relations. As far as I can see, there was no family relationship between Hannah and Mary, at least not a close one. It's telling that, when Hannah made a bequest to a relative in her will, she named the relationship – 'daughter of my cousin', 'my cousin', etc. – unless it was someone who either had the surname Beswick (e.g. Edmund Beswick of Blackley) or was born with the surname Beswick (e.g. Ann wife of Thomas Apperly of Ross in the County of Hereford).[14] Mary Greame got no such explanation, being simply described as 'Mary Greame of Salford, spinster'.

There are two other unexplained spinsters in Hannah's will: Elizabeth Wood of Manchester and Sarah Jenkinson of Manchester. Elizabeth got a monogrammed silver meat spoon and 'a couple of silver candlesticks', and Sarah got an income for life, but only if she completed a very specific condition of the will. Mary Greame, though, not only got the tenancy of Cheetwood Hall (including all of Hannah's household and furniture) for the rest of her life and some personal effects, but also £200 or whatever it cost to complete the task Hannah set her at the end of her will. This was clearly an important relationship, but it doesn't appear to have been a familial one.

Mary Greame was born in Skircoat, near Halifax, to John and Martha Greame (née Earnshaw).[15] She had a brother, John, and a sister, Ann. If the date on Mary's gravestone is correct, she was born in 1718, making her forty years old when Hannah died. It should be noted that, although Mary's family was from Halifax, Hannah calls her 'Mary Greame of Salford'.

In 1743, Mary's sister Ann married Thomas Gorton of Salford. Thomas was the son of John Gorton, a man who claimed to have been born in the Fylde at some point around 1690 and to have worked as a miller's servant. One day, when John – nicknamed John-o-potbo – was delivering flour near Preston, he saw a man acting suspiciously near some turf. When the man had gone, John went to investigate and discovered that the stranger had been burying treasure in the ground. It was, you see, 1715, the year of the *first* Jacobite rebellion. So frightened was this man of the *Old* Pretender's army marching across Lancashire, that he buried his treasures instead of seeing them taken. Unfortunately for this terrified man, John-o-potbo found them before he could return to collect them, and the miller's servant took his new-found riches to Manchester.[16]

I include this story partly because of its remarkable similarity to the 'Legend of Birchen Bower'. Just as Madame Beswick was so scared of the Pretender's army in the '45 that she buried her gold at Birchen Bower, this anonymous Preston man was so scared in the '15 that he buried his gold in the turf. Joe at Tamer's found Madame Beswick's gold and took it to Manchester; John-o-potbo found the Preston gold and also headed to Manchester.

The John (or Joan)-o-potbo story was written by John Higson, and it was included in his book, *The Gorton Historical Recorder*, in 1852. According to folklore historian Simon Young: 'Born to a poor family, raised without an education, Higson became, through hard-work and talent one of the most exciting Lancashire folklore writers of his generation, and got to be friends with some of the most influential county authors of his day.'[17] That description has a lot in common with the biography of James Dronsfield of Hollinwood, who wrote the original 'Legend of Birchen Bower' article in 1869, introducing readers to Madame Beswick's buried gold and the lucky Joe at Tamer's. John Higson's book begins with an introduction to Gorton, a township to the south-east of Manchester, in the 1850s:

> Let us compare the past with the present. What a change has come over the scene! The ancient trees are felled, the *lanes* are being superseded by *roads*, and are assuming modernised appellations; pack-horses are fled; their place is supplied by railway engines, for we have now two railways passing through the township, besides a canal, and an excellent new road to Manchester, &c.[18]

This reads a lot like a description of the changes felt in Hollinwood in the 1860s, though Hollinwood only had the one railway line. Now, I'm not saying that James Dronsfield knowingly lifted the story of John-o-potbo and the '15 from Higson and translated it into Joe at Tamer's and the '45, but I have to note the coincidence of two writers, both trying to capture the Lancashire character of particular areas on the outskirts of Manchester in times gone by, including a strikingly similar story about Jacobite panic in their accounts. What's really weird is that the two people featured in the stories were real, and that the son of John-o-potbo was actually a close friend of Madame Beswick. That bit, I can't account for.

The other reason I mention the 'legend' of John Gorton's wealth is to show that Thomas Gorton of Salford (and, later, Gorton Hall) was about as nouveau bourgeois as they come. Not only had Thomas Gorton's father not been born a gentleman, he'd actually been (according to legend) a servant. Leaving aside – once again – the question of buried treasure, more 'serious' records show that John Gorton, father of Thomas, was not a member of the ancestral Gortons of Gorton, but rather a man who arrived in the township cash-rich (however he acquired that cash) and ready to buy property. In 1722, he bought Gorton Hall itself, establishing his family there as if it was their ancestral home. By 1732, John-o-potbo was John Gorton, gentleman.

Thomas was John's youngest son, and he was a successful businessman and merchant. Although Thomas held a number of titles, he's listed in some records as a 'flower-seller'. In 1767, Thomas got in on Manchester's auricula boom. Auriculas – hardy perennials that are part of the genus Primula – had been grown in the Manchester area from around 1720, but by the 1760s, the town was 'particularly known' for them. Thomas advertised five auriculas: 'Earl of Chatham' and 'Liberty' (one guinea each), 'Countess of Chatham', 'Lord Cambden' and 'Bright Flora' (half a guinea).[19] It wasn't exactly tulip mania, but Thomas boasted that his Liberty was 'one of the best Cheyne Flowers that ever appeared; its Stem and Trussing is the same as the Dutch Flower Flora Perfecta; its Eye is extraordinary, and will stand a Month in Bloom, and dye one of the best blues ever seen in an Auricula'.[20] As well as being a florist and a businessman, Thomas would go on to be a boroughreeve of Salford and warden of the Gorton Chapel. When he died in 1789, he was described as 'a Gentleman, in every Respect, whether of a public or private Character, a very worthy and upright Man; a kind Parent, a steady Friend, and a sincere Christian'.[21] He was the very model of early modern social mobility.

When Thomas married Ann Greame in 1743, he also apparently acquired her sister. Mary Greame was around twenty-five years old when her sister got married, and she was a spinster. Her parents were dead, and so she went to live in Salford with her new brother-in-law, rather than staying in Exley (near Skircoat) with her brother. Perhaps Thomas had hopes of finding a husband for his sister-in-law, but these hopes were to be dashed. Mary Greame would spend the next twenty-four years of her life as a confirmed spinster.

I don't know how Hannah became friends with Thomas Gorton's family, but she definitely did. In her will, she left Ann, Thomas's wife, her finest silver platter (to which we'll return shortly), her brocaded silk nightgown (valued at £2 10s) and six yards of Brussels lace (valued at £3). She also left Thomas and Ann's daughter Margaret the sum of fifty pounds. When the will was challenged by Thomas Robinson in 1761, an inventory was drawn up, including all payments that had been made out of the estate since Hannah's death. One of these was for £10 to Thomas Gorton, 'for his expenses and trouble in transacting all the affairs relating to the deceased's will'.

The biggest bequest to the family, though, was to Mary. Hannah set Mary up with a home for the rest of her life, as well as material goods and money. However, Hannah also placed a huge amount of trust in Mary, making her executor of the will and one of the people responsible for ensuring her last wishes were carried out. Mary was certainly younger than Hannah, by twenty-four years, but she wasn't a young woman like Esther Robinson.

In the nine years following Hannah's death, Mary would indeed make her home at Cheetwood Hall. But things would change in 1767, when – in a surprise turn of events – Mary finally got married, at the age of fifty, to a lawyer from Halifax.

Richard Hopwood was a childless widower in 1767, as his first wife, Mary Morton, had died in 1765. It's possible that Richard Hopwood is the 'Mr Hopwood the attorney' who was paid 10s for services after Hannah's death, and if this is the case, I'd suggest the 'services' might relate to Hannah's property in Yorkshire. Certainly, Mary's brother-in-law supported the marriage, as he agreed to a £10,000 marriage bond to ensure their marriage licence. A marriage bond was an agreement made, usually by the groom and a close relative of the bride, with the vicar or priest conducting the marriage that guaranteed, if it turned out the couple were not legally allowed to marry, the bondsmen would pay the agreed fee as a fine to the church. It was an alternative to posting banns, and it was the favoured route of people with financial means. £10,000 is a remarkably high bond, as it was more common at the time to see hundreds, rather than thousands, of pounds being pledged for marriage licences. This is probably a reflection of the high status and wealth of the bondsmen, but also the fact that the couple were older, and that one of them had been married before.

After five decades of spinsterhood, and the relative economic freedom this allowed, Mary was now a wife, with her legal identity subsumed into that of her husband. She moved out of Hannah's house and into Richard Hopwood's, surrendering certain documents to Hannah's other executor, Charles White, when she did so.[22]

It's hard to rein in your imagination when thinking about Mary's marriage to Richard Hopwood. Maybe Mary had always been in love with Richard, but he was married to someone else. When his first wife died, he turned to his old friend for comfort and the two were finally married. Or maybe, Mary was indeed a confirmed spinster, living at the home of a woman who had been her close companion for fifteen years, until her brother-in-law had suggested a more 'respectable' relationship with a wealthy widower.

The option you favour for the reason behind Mary's marriage will colour your response to what happened next. Richard Hopwood died in 1769, less than two years after his second marriage. Mary Hopwood (née Greame) lived for another twenty years, as a rich widow with the economic independence that identity conferred. When Mary made her own will in 1789, she left a substantial property portfolio, including at least one property that she appears to have bought herself after her husband's death, and several large monetary bequests that were almost all to her own nieces and nephews. There is only one person with the surname Hopwood in Mary's will, and that's the wife of her husband's nephew. The rest of her estate goes to Ann, Henry, Thomas and Frances (the children of her brother John) with John Dyson and John Holden (her sister Ann's sons-in-law) as executors. The furniture she brought to Halifax from Cheetwood was left to her niece Ann Greame.

* * *

The phrase 'sundry odd things' appears in the inventory of Hannah's estate made in 1761 when Thomas Robinson brought his lawsuit after the death of his son Joshua. It's at the end of a list of Hannah's 'wearing apparel' and likely denotes odd accessories that were considered to be of little value. But Hannah's will contains other sundry odd things that are intriguing – maybe even revealing. Specifically, there's a large silver plate, some funeral expenses, and a very particular set of instructions for a trio of spinsters.

Let's start with the plate. One of Hannah's bequests to Ann Gorton was a 'silver waiter' (i.e. a large platter). There are a number of instructions about silverware in the will, and these seem to be small gifts to women of Hannah's acquaintance, which isn't very unusual. However, in the case of this particular platter, Hannah leaves it to Ann, but only in the event that it isn't 'taken for a herriott'. This needs a bit of explanation.

A 'herriott' or 'heriot' was an archaic form of death duty owed to the lord of the manor after the death of a copyholder. It derives from an early medieval custom – the word comes from the Old English 'heregeat' or 'war gear' – by which the king would be presented with a set of arms or a war horse on the death of a nobleman. The custom developed in the later Middle Ages, becoming the practice of 'feudal relief' or inheritance tax, in which the lord of the manor would be owed a high value item, usually a horse, cow or ox, as a 'fine' when one of his villeins (tenants) died.

By the eighteenth century, heriots were part of copyhold tenure. On the death of a tenant, the best 'chattel' (possession) or beast was taken by their landlord as death duty. Other forms of death duty had started to be introduced by this point, including probate duty (part of the Stamps Act 1694) which imposed a charge (payable to the government, rather than the landlord) for any probate on an estate larger than £20. Later in the eighteenth century, 'legacy duty' would be introduced, a forerunner to modern inheritance tax. There were some who lamented the demise of the heriot and its replacement with legacy duty, as the former was taken out of the personal goods of the deceased, while the latter was taken out of the inheritance of the heir.

Hannah held lands in copyhold from the Duke of Devonshire who, at the time of her death, was one of the richest and most powerful men in the country. William Cavendish, 4th Duke of Devonshire, was the (nominal) prime minister in 1756–57, the man who paid Capability

Brown to design the famous gardens at Chatsworth, and a great-great-great-great-great-grandfather of King Charles III. He was also the lord of the manor to whom Hannah's copyhold lands had to be surrendered on her death.

Hannah's instructions about the silver platter show a shrewd awareness of the legalities of her last will and testament. She reveals an understanding of the status of copyhold tenure, and she makes things easier for her executors by signalling the high value 'chattel' that should be set aside in case of death duties. It's a sensible and rational instruction, and it's one of the aspects of her will that makes you think Robert Radclyffe and John Saxon were absolutely right to step back and leave John Beswick's estate under his sister's control.

And yet, there's something a little odd about Hannah's instructions over the platter. Firstly, it's not the highest value item in her estate, as the inventory reveals the silver candlesticks and a gold watch were worth more. Secondly, she first states who she *wants* to give it to, and then notes that it might be taken by the Duke. It all feels a bit pointed, as though she is saying that her friend Ann, who likely knew the platter from spending time with Hannah at Cheetwood, is the rightful recipient, but she had to be aware of the potential for aristocratic seizure. And it's hard not to notice that Hannah gave the platter, which she had expressly stated was good enough to be taken as a heriot by the Duke of Devonshire himself, to the wife of a nouveau-riche florist from Salford.

A nice interpretation is that Hannah was revealing how much she valued her friend – Ann was deserving of the highest value item in Hannah's possession. However, it's hard not to also wonder whether Hannah is throwing just the tiniest bit of shade on the Duke of Devonshire, or on the feudal system of tenure that he represents. There's just a hint of an implication here that Hannah's actual wishes might be undermined by an archaic practice through which a duke, who had absolutely no need for additional silverware, could swoop in and take your biggest plate.

In case you're curious, Ann got the big plate. The Duke of Devonshire took his heriot in cash – £15 15s to be precise. This wasn't such a bad deal in the end, as the silver platter was only worth £8. And it was substantially less of an outlay than the 'fine' imposed by the Earl of Derby for adding Hannah's heirs to the lease on Cheetwood (another form of death duty), which was a whopping £255 1s 5d.

Hannah's big silver plate is a rather charming curiosity, and it's not one that's ever really been noted by people who have studied her will. This is hardly surprising, because apart from Stephen Baxter's interest in Mrs Gilbert Gorton's silk nightgown and some passing concern about the ownership of Birchen Bower, Hannah's will has only ever been examined for evidence of her desire to be mummified. And we already know that her will says nothing about mummification.

Or does it?

* * *

Like her brother and her father – and almost every other person who has ever left a will – Hannah's last will and testament makes provision for funeral expenses. When someone dies, unless they leave specific instructions to the contrary, the expense of their funeral comes out of the estate before it's divided up between the heirs. Both Hannah's father and her brother acknowledged this in their wills, stating that funeral expenses should be paid out before the estate was granted to their rightful heir.

Hannah's will sort of says this too, but she was a bit clearer about what it meant. She left the amount of £400 to her 'executrixes' (meaning Mary and Esther, but not Charles White) to 'defray the expenses of my funeral' and then, if there was any money left over, to distribute to her relatives on her father's side at Mary and Esther's own discretion. In fact, she stated explicitly that Mary and Esther were not to be questioned by anyone as to how they distributed any surplus. This final statement is a palimpsest – whatever was originally written in the will was erased, scraped off the vellum, and then overwritten with the new instruction. This could've been a simple mistake, but it's a bit of a coincidence that a scribal error happened right at the moment when a woman – who would end up mummified and put in a museum – was describing her post-mortem wishes. No, I think that the will had to be corrected because of the unorthodox nature of the instructions. Hannah's lawyer, Dauntesey Smith, was ensuring that the wording was unequivocal and legally binding. The resulting instructions, including the very high sum of money laid out for the funeral, was described by one Lancashire County archivist in the 1930s, Fred Booth, as 'very unusual'.

A lot of work went into creating Hannah's will. As well as Dauntesey Smith, who drew up the document, 'Lawyer Kenyon' and 'Lawyer Lee' gave advice and a 'Lawyer Wilbraham' gave an opinion (all of whom were paid for this service from the estate). 'Mr Hopwood the attorney' was also paid for undefined services, and Thomas Gorton received £10 for expenses related to carrying out the deceased's wishes.

It's quite a simple fact: £400 is far too high an amount for a normal funeral in 1758. That's what Fred Booth spotted when he looked at the will in the 1930s, and that's what we'll have to come back to later in the story.

For now, we need to spot the last 'odd thing', the instruction Hannah gave to Mary, Esther and Sarah Jenkinson at the end of her will. You'll remember that each of the women would be set up for life by the terms of Hannah's final wishes – Esther got the house on King Street, Mary got Cheetwood Hall and Sarah got a lifetime income – but only if they did one last thing for Hannah.[23]

The three spinsters, Mary, Esther and Sarah, had to live together at Cheetwood Hall for two years after Hannah's death.

Now that is odd.

10
Oil of lavender

A lot of things changed in Hannah's lifetime. Even the calendar changed when she was in her late fifties – the United Kingdom (as it was by then) adopted the Gregorian calendar in September 1752, eliding eleven days of the year in the process. Was it weird for Hannah to go to bed on Wednesday 2 September and wake up on Thursday 14 September? Or was it more of hassle, as she had to ensure that the rents on her property and payments from those in debt to her were deferred for eleven days?[1]

But, for a story that partly revolves around a woman's relationship with a doctor, it's the changes to the medical profession that are of most significance. In earlier chapters, I've used the word 'surgeon' a lot, so let's start there. What is a surgeon?

Surgery is the process of manually, or with the use of instruments, reaching into a patient's body to treat disease or injury. In its early form, it was practised alongside bone-setting as way of repairing and remedying afflictions. In medieval and early modern England, the most common practitioners of surgery were barbers, who were well placed (due to the instruments they used and the hand-eye coordination they needed) to carry out procedures like pulling teeth, bloodletting and wound-dressing that were common forms of surgery. However, there were also medical surgeons around at this time, who qualified after serving an apprenticeship with an established surgeon. Often, these medical surgeons were performing the same set of procedures as barber-surgeons (though, one assumes, without offering haircuts as well), and so it's no surprise that in 1540, the Guild of Surgeons (representing medical surgeons) merged with the Worshipful Company of Barbers to form the Company of Barber-Surgeons.[2]

Surgeons were not physicians. Physicians were medical doctors who, after academic training rather than apprenticeship, were qualified to study, diagnose and treat disease. Early modern physicians were often involved in scientific study – for instance, biology or epidemiology – rather than the physical procedures for manipulating the human body employed by surgeons. This is a somewhat simplistic distinction between two types of doctors – and it doesn't take into account the existence of other medical professionals, such as midwives – because there isn't space here for a full history of the medical profession.

What matters for Hannah's story is that, for quite some time, physician and surgeon had been different professions, requiring different training.

But all that was about to change.

In 1745, the barbers and surgeons officially went their separate ways, and an Act of Parliament was passed to formally distinguish the two professions. The surgeons were to form the Company of Surgeons, which would later go on to be the (Royal) College of Surgeons, a body that not only represented but also licensed qualified practitioners. Barbers continued to practise surgical procedures, but – as time would tell – they would gain a reputation for being unqualified, old-fashioned or downright dangerous.[3]

As medical practice developed, the role of the surgeon became less distinct from the role of the physician. This was particularly apparent when it came to the study of anatomy. Knowledge of human anatomy was vital for the surgeon, who had to know how the body worked in order to manipulate and treat it; however, it was also a key aspect of the scientific and academic training of the physician, who also had to know how (and why) the body worked. If a physician required formal academic training in order to understand human anatomy, did a surgeon not need this as well? And how should this academic training be provided?

Again, this is not a history of medicine, but rather an overview of the historical context for the story of Hannah Beswick. In order to see the relevance of this background, it's probably best that we look at a specific example of medical and surgical training in the eighteenth century. Let's look at Dr Charles White.

* * *

Charles White was born in Manchester in 1728. His father, Thomas White, was a physician, having been licensed by the College of Physicians in 1733, after examination by members of the college, including its president, Hans Sloane.[4] In his medical practice, however, Thomas White focused on surgery and midwifery, showing that, by the 1730s, a licensed physician was qualified to practise medicine more broadly.

Charles White followed in his father's footsteps, and his training reveals a lot about how medical education was changing in eighteenth-century England. In his teens, White was apprenticed to his father in Manchester, introducing him to both surgery and midwifery. In later life, White would claim to have had experience of 'lying-in' (the treatment of pregnant women) before he'd turned eighteen.[5]

However, to become a licensed doctor like his father, White also needed academic training. For this, he had to travel to London, where he would study under William Hunter, a man considered to be the leading anatomist of his day.

William Hunter was born in East Kilbride, south-east of Glasgow, in 1718. After studying divinity at the University of Glasgow, he embarked on his medical training under the tutelage of eminent physician William Cullen. However, Hunter had needed practical training as well as academic training, and so he also travelled to London, becoming a resident pupil of obstetrician and anatomist William Smellie at St George's Hospital. Once qualified, Hunter followed Smellie in teaching in anatomy and obstetrics, giving courses at London hospitals, as well as private courses on dissection and surgery.

White attended Hunter's lectures while in London, and he studied alongside Hunter's younger brother John, who would go on to be a prominent anatomist and surgeon in his own right. We've met the Hunter brothers earlier in this story, of course, as one of them (likely William) embalmed the body of Maria van Butchell for display in her husband's dental surgery. John Hunter would go on to dissect the body of Charles Byrne, known as the 'Irish Giant', in 1783, against the man's wishes. The skeleton of Charles Byrne is still held by the Hunterian Museum at the Royal College of Surgeons in London, despite calls for it to be removed and buried.

After attending lectures in London, White would go on to study for a short time in Edinburgh, before returning to Manchester to complete his training with his father. It was not until 1762 – by which time White was a prominent member of Manchester's medical elite, having helped to found the Manchester Infirmary – that White actually received a qualification, a diploma of Member of the Company of Surgeons.[6] The fact that White was a member of the Company of Surgeons, while his father was licensed by the College of Physicians is significant. The two men were engaged in literally the same medical practice in Manchester, and so this is a very clear example of how the relationship between physician and surgeon was changing in the eighteenth century.

So, what sort of teaching did White receive from Hunter when he was in London? The separation of the barbers and the surgeons in 1745 had resulted in the removal of certain by-laws restricting the dissection of human bodies. This meant that 'private' lecturers (i.e. practitioners not employed or directed by the Company of Surgeons) could offer classes in 'practical anatomy' at either their own residences or in purpose-built lecture theatres. Simon Chaplin has described Hunter as part of 'the new breed of entrepreneurial surgeon-anatomist', whose insistence on teaching anatomy through the dissection of corpses, rather than the delineation of the human body through diagrams and illustrations, radically changed the medical curriculum in London.[7] Chaplin captures the impact of this change:

> Their [the surgeon-anatomists] courses, together with the clinical instruction offered in charitable hospitals, were the main reasons why so many would-be practitioners flocked to London. Over 10,000 young men signed up as hospital pupils in London between 1750 and 1815, and it is likely that many more attended extra-mural lectures.[8]

Extra-mural here means outside of the medical curriculum, and so it includes lectures that were open to the general public. For instance, one anatomist, William Cheselden, advertised his lecture course to: 'Those who study anatomy for their Entertainment, or to qualify Themselves for the Knowledge of physick or surgery, and not for such as wou'd be critically knowing in the most minute Parts.'[9] Later in the eighteenth century, surgeon John Sheldon (the man who reportedly kept Miss Johnson's embalmed body in a case under his bed) advertised a course where 'Gentlemen who are desirous of merely visiting the Dissections, without operating' could attend his lectures for a subscription of five guineas.[10]

The references here to 'entertainment' and people 'visiting dissections' conjure up a somewhat ghoulish picture, but it's important to remember that this was an integral part of medical training in the eighteenth century. When Richard Kay of Walmersley – a man who, as his rather mundane diary reveals, was about as far from a ghoulish devotee of public dissections as you could get – undertook his medical qualification in the early 1740s, he travelled to London to attend lectures at hospital theatres and anatomy halls, given by, among others, William Smellie.[11] Like Charles White, Richard Kay would return to his hometown after receiving this education, ready to put his academic knowledge into practice.

The rise in practical anatomy lectures in both 'public' settings (those run by the Company of Surgeons) and 'private' (those offered by surgeon-anatomists on a 'freelance' basis, either for hospitals or in private venues) meant that resources had to be found. Students weren't in short supply, so new buildings had to be adapted or constructed in order to house the growing audiences for dissections.

And, obviously, there had to be bodies to dissect.

The Murder Act 1751 (1752) was an act of parliament governing, as you might have guessed, the punishments for murder. Prior to this act being passed, a judge giving a death sentence had the power to order that the body of the executed prisoner be dissected. When the Murder Act was passed, dissection became mandatory. The Act stated explicitly that execution wasn't enough of a deterrent and so, 'some further terror and peculiar mark of infamy [should] be added to the punishment of death'. The bodies of people hanged for murder could not be lawfully buried. They had to either be gibbeted (put on public display in chains) or publicly dissected. The Company of Surgeons was required *by law* to carry out anatomical dissections on the bodies of those hanged for murder, and students like Charles White would attend these dissections as part of their training.

This use of the bodies of executed criminals in public dissection wasn't uncontroversial. In 1749, shortly before the Murder Act was passed but when the practice of judges ordering dissection as part of a death sentence was well established, the so-called Tyburn Riot occurred, in which the friends and families of executed prisoners rushed the scaffold to retrieve the bodies of their loved ones before they could be sent to the anatomists.[12] There were other incidents of this nature, with relatives of convicted murderers fighting with the beadles of the Company of Surgeons to stop the deceased from receiving this 'peculiar mark of infamy'.

We're linking back up to an earlier chapter now, as the practice laid out by the Murder Act would expand to include the bodies of people who died in workhouses, asylums and infirmaries who had been sent for a medical post-mortem, which would in turn lead to the Cholera Riots of the early 1830s.[13] And it's also worth noting – though the crimes of William Burke and William Hare, and the grave-robbing tactics of the 'resurrection men' would make this abundantly clear – there simply weren't enough people being convicted of murder to supply the anatomy halls (perhaps the Murder Act *did* work as a deterrent). Other methods were needed to ensure a supply of cadavers for practical anatomy classes, particularly given the continued rise in the numbers of medical students.

Welcome to the old body-snatching days.

* * *

Although William Hunter was the man who helped to lead the new style of anatomy teaching in eighteenth-century London, it was his brother John who is most associated with the 'art' of public dissection. In her biography of John Hunter, Wendy Moore suggests that the man 'dissected human bodies in unprecedented numbers'.[14] In addition to this, John Hunter was the anatomist most connected to the resurrection men of Georgian London, even going so far as to openly admit to grave-robbing in one of his casebooks: 'we got a stout Man for the Muscles from St George's ground'.[15]

However, as both the Hunters knew, practical anatomy was taught through more than just dissection. Specimens of various human body parts were needed to demonstrate the 'minute parts' of anatomical structure. An anatomist conducting a dissection might choose to retain a body part of particular interest – a malformed joint, for instance, or an enlarged organ – and then preserve it for teaching purposes at a later date. These might be 'wet' preparations (specimens kept in jars, suspended in liquid preservatives) or 'dry' preparations (bone fragments or dried body parts). Chaplin suggests these were 'manifestly useful objects' for anatomy teachers, as they didn't decay like a cadaver and could be used time and again.[16] Teachers such as William Hunter taught their students how to prepare these preparations correctly, and they encouraged prospective medical men to build up their own collections of preparations. Or a medical cabinet, if you will.

John Hunter built up an extensive cabinet of preparations during his career, which would become the 'extraordinary collection of specimens' from which the Hunterian Museum at the Royal College of Surgeons would grow.[17] When the collection was first lodged with the College of Surgeons, it was estimated that there were around 14,000 specimens; however, only 3,000 of these still survive, as the museum was a casualty of the Blitz, partially destroyed by an incendiary bomb in 1941. Some of the surviving specimens are still on display at the museum, as human body parts over 100 years are not governed by the Human Tissue Act 2004 and so currently have no restrictions on their use or display, but it is no longer possible to see the more notorious specimens that were housed at the museum in the nineteenth century. The bodies of Maria van Butchell and Miss Johnson were destroyed in the 1941 bomb, and the skeleton of Charles Byrne has been removed from display until a decision can be made about its future in the collection.

Another prolific eighteenth-century collector of anatomical specimens was John Sheldon. As we've already seen, the travel writer Barthélemy Faujas de Saint-Fond described a visit to Sheldon's cabinet in the late 1790s, which he described as 'one of the finest anatomical cabinets in existence'. It was here that Faujas de Saint-Fond would encounter the body of Miss Johnson, the supposed mistress of the doctor. If we return to Sheldon's cabinet with the teaching of anatomy in mind, we might question why such a specimen would be included in a collection intended for academic study and demonstrative purpose. What use could a mummified woman be, other than as a curiosity?

In his account of Sheldon's cabinet, Faujas de Saint-Fond offers a brief explanation of how the body of Miss Johnson was preserved:

> He injected several parts of the body with strong spirits of wine, saturated with camphire [henna], and mixed with a small quantity of turpentine.
>
> The skin was prepared and tanned, as it were, with finely powdered alum, rubbed on with the hand. The intestines were taken out, and covered with a varnish, composed of a mixture of camphire, and the common rosin. The same thing was done to all the internal parts of the body, which were afterwards passed over with alum.
>
> Sheldon assured me, that pulverized camphire, mixed with rosin, formed an excellent composition for preserving the flesh, and other soft parts. After having placed all the viscera thus prepared in the body, he then injected the crural artery with a strong solution of camphire, in rectified spirit.
>
> Wishing afterwards to imitate the natural tint of the skin of the face, a coloured injection was pushed through the carotides, to produce that effect.
>
> In this state of things the body was placed in the table of which I have spoken; but within a double case of timber [...] The inner bottom was covered with calcined chalk, to the thickness of one inch, in order to absorb all humidity. Upon this bed the body was extended. The box, or case, was then carefully shut up, to secure the body from the impression of the external air.
>
> The box was not opened until five years after the preparation was made. It was then observed to be in the same state of preservation in which it was first enclosed. No mark of decay appeared, and no insect had introduced itself near the body.[18]

The method being outlined here follows William Hunter's technique for embalming the human body, which was a development of (and progression from) earlier techniques practised by anatomists in Paris.

According to Thomas Joseph Pettigrew, writing in 1834, William Hunter's anatomy lectures often ended with some instruction on making anatomical preparations. It was in this way that Hunter first advanced his proposed method for embalming an entire cadaver. Hunter's method, as laid out by Pettigrew, looks very similar to the method Faujas de Saint-Fond attributed to Sheldon. Viscera are removed, and then various solutions are injected into the veins and blood vessels of the corpse:

> The method he proposed was to throw into the blood-vessels, in the most minute manner he was able, an injection composed of essential oil of turpentine, in which a small proportion of Venice turpentine had been dissolved. To this he added different proportions of oil of camomile and oil of lavender, and coloured the whole with vermilion. This fluid having been forced into the large arteries with such power and continuance that even the skin exhibited a red appearance, the body was allowed to remain some hours undisturbed, to admit of the mixture thoroughly impregnating it.[19]

Finally, the body was placed 'upon a bed of plaster of Paris, by which all moisture would be absorbed': 'The coffin was to be closed up, and at the expiration of four years opened, and should the dessication [*sic*] of the body be imperfect, another bed of gypsum was to be added to complete the process.'[20]

I don't quote this description for macabre or ghoulish purposes. It's important to know what Hunter was proposing, and what Sheldon replicated. While there's no doubt that anatomists such as the Hunters and Sheldon were trying out techniques and procedures for prestige, fame and notoriety, they were also scientists. They were trying to discover everything they could about the human form, and to develop ways of passing this knowledge on to others (even if some of those others were only there for 'entertainment').

Look closely (ignore the turpentine and oil of lavender for a moment) and you'll see that Hunter and Sheldon's techniques both involve arterial or venous injection. Unlike earlier techniques for embalming that involved making large incisions in the body, Hunter's method used the body's own circulatory system to introduce preservative chemicals into the tissue. In this, he was following the principles laid out by William Harvey in the previous century. Harvey was the first known physician to fully describe the circulatory system in detail, including the properties of veins and arteries, and it is only because of his scientific discoveries that Hunter was able to work out a technique for preserving an entire cadaver.

The problem is, you can only embalm someone once. The act of embalming might be a great opportunity to demonstrate the circulatory system and the preservative properties of certain chemicals, but once the box is reopened and the results revealed (to the wonder of your audience), you're just left with a corpse, and one that you can't bury, because it's several years since the person actually died. The embalmed body is not a 'manifestly useful object'. It's little more than a curiosity.

This might explain why, when he visited Sheldon's cabinet in the late eighteenth century, Faujas de Saint-Fond spent hours poring over diagrams and engravings of the lymphatic system, but only a short time examining the body of Miss Johnson. The method of embalming was of interest to him – he recounted it in full in his narrative – but the actual material specimen was something curious, but also distasteful. This is also seen in the case of Maria van Butchell. The continued display of the woman's body in the museum revealed, not the techniques and scientific knowledge behind its preservation, but rather the limitations of Hunter's technique. Although the body might have been in a perfect state of preservation when the box was first opened, it degraded over time to become 'a wretched mockery of a once lovely woman'.

* * *

Charles White returned to Manchester, armed with all the knowledge his London education had provided, ready to join his father's practice on King Street. However, he was clearly frustrated by the fact that, in order to obtain his medical education, he had had to leave Manchester.

Again, we're linking back to a previous chapter here, as I've already described how White tried to further the teaching of anatomy and surgery in late eighteenth-century Manchester through his work with the College of Arts and Sciences.

White's attempts at creating a scholarly environment in which anatomy could be studied in Manchester was important for the town, as well as for the man himself. As should be abundantly clear from earlier chapters, eighteenth-century and early nineteenth-century Manchester had ambitions to be more than a provincial town. Just as St Ann's Square was constructed to rival the fashionable squares of London and Bath, White's anatomy lectures were designed to match those in the capital, including bringing in 'guest speakers' from London and Edinburgh. It would be some time before a Mancunian institution had the authority to award actual medical degrees, but White's teaching appears to have been modelled on the anatomy lectures he had attended in London (the metropolis) and Edinburgh (the Athens of the North).

For that, White needed demonstration materials, cadavers both for dissection and for preparation. It's clear that this wasn't a problem, though, as over the decades Charles White was able to build up an anatomical cabinet, containing both human and animal specimens. When his father Thomas retired in 1776, White continued to practise at the King Street house, inviting fellow surgeons and prospective medical students to view his surgical operations, and showing his anatomical cabinet to interested parties. White also took his preparations out to lectures at other venues. At a meeting of the Manchester Lit and Phil in November 1784, White exhibited a thigh bone from his collection, where it was compared with elephant thigh bones from the cabinets of William Hunter, Hans Sloane and Ashton Lever.[21]

As well as practising surgery and midwifery, and giving lectures, White also continued his academic study of the human body. The outcome of this is very much a game of two halves.

On the one hand, White was an exponent of a polygenist theory of race, believing that different races constituted different species or subspecies. His book, *An Account of the Regular Gradation in Man, and in Different Animals and Vegetables; and From the Former to the Latter*, was published in 1799, and, according to the author's preface, was inspired by hearing John Hunter give a lecture on the 'Gradation of Skulls' in Manchester, at the Lying-In Hospital the previous year.[22] In this book, White offers up 'evidence' of the physiological difference between races, including a large number of measurements, to support his hypothesis. This book makes for unpleasant reading, particularly when he describes the process of measuring a 'negro' at the 'lunatic asylum' in Liverpool, to prove that his forearms were a different size to the European average, and when he writes about the genitals of both male and female subjects he has measured. His argument throughout is, to put it bluntly, that people of African descent are closer to apes in their physiology than Europeans are. Surprisingly, perhaps, White begins his book by stating that he doesn't want to see the 'facts' he will lay out being used as a justification for 'the pernicious practice of enslaving mankind, which he wishes to see abolished throughout the world'.[23]

Nevertheless, theories such as those put forward by White would indeed be used as justification for slavery, and we can see echoes of this type of argument in the treatment of, for instance, Julia Pastrana and Saartje Baartman in the nineteenth century. Charles Darwin wrote about Julia Pastana in his book *The Variation of Animals and Plants Under Domestication*, commenting on her 'gorilla-like appearance', and Saartje Baartman was marketed, in her lifetime, as the 'missing link'. Saartje Baartman was known as the 'Hottentot Venus', and in his 1799 book White discusses the genitals and breasts of 'the Hottentot women', stating '[n]o European white woman, however, in any age or climate, was ever known to have a breast of such description'.[24]

On the other hand, White was an expert in obstetrics and a successful 'man-midwife'. In 1773, he published what is considered to be his most significant work, his *Treatise on the Management of Pregnant and Lying-In Women*. In this work, White sets out his explanation for high rates of maternal mortality and disease. He describes the usual practice for delivering a baby, pointing out that the conditions in which childbirth took place were themselves the cause of sickness and death. He proposed new practices, including a fresh flow of air to the room, regular handwashing for those attending the birth, clean towels, bed linen and instruments. He also argued for women to be allowed to move and stand upright after giving birth, rather than being bedbound in a horizontal position in the days following childbirth. Finally, he suggested that any woman showing signs of fever should be isolated for ten days, to avoid the spread of illness.

All this might seem like common sense, but White's proposed practice was radical. As a result, he entirely eradicated puerperal fever on the wards of the Infirmary and, later, the Lying-In Hospital. This illness – also known as 'the doctor's plague' – was the most common cause of maternal mortality in the early eighteenth century and, by the beginning of the nineteenth century, White had saved the lives of thousands of women. White's book – which was published in five editions, reprinted in America, and translated into German and French – has been described as a 'revolution in midwifery', and White was proud to state that, in all of the normal labours he had attended, he had 'never lost a mother from puerperal sepsis'.[25]

White's career shows a desire to replicate certain elements of metropolitan medical practice, including teaching, in a more provincial setting. This included, of course, the 'collections-based pedagogy that dominated the age'.[26] White's medical cabinet was first housed at his house on the corner of King Street and Cross Street. 'Dr *White*'s Anatomical Museum, in Cross-street' was clearly well enough known in the 1780s to appear in an advertisement for the College of Arts and Sciences as a place to buy tickets for lectures. This was the cabinet that Thomas de Quincey visited as a young man, when it apparently contained both the skeleton of a highwayman and the embalmed body of one of White's patients.

When White moved from King Street to Sale Priory, he tried to sell part of his anatomical cabinet to the infirmary, offering a selection of specimens to the hospital for the sum of £226. This offer was rejected, and White instead gave his museum to the Lying-In Hospital, and it was opened to the public 'the first Monday in every month, at eleven o'clock, for the reception of ladies; and at one, for the reception of gentlemen'.[27] White's museum at the Lying-In Hospital had 285 exhibits in total, including a corroded human liver, the skeleton of a foetus and a chicken with two heads.[28]

The body of Hannah Beswick wasn't included in White's museum at the Lying-In Hospital. The assumption is that he took it to Sale Priory when he moved there in the late 1790s. My guess is that the specimen, as with other embalmed bodies, was no longer a 'manifestly useful object', and so had no purpose as a teaching tool. It was – as we saw in the first half of the book – simply a curiosity, and so it was stored somewhere at White's house (probably not on the roof) until the end of his life.

White left no instructions about the body of Hannah Beswick in his will. It is believed that he gave it to another Manchester doctor, Thomas Ollier, who eventually deposited it with the Natural History Society, but no records of this survive. All we know is that, by 1834, it was on display in the King Street museum.

To quote Harry Ludlam, some small mysteries remain. Not least, how did Hannah end up getting embalmed in the first place? She wasn't a convicted murderer, taken from the scaffold by a beadle under the provision of the Murder Act. She certainly wasn't the inmate of a workhouse or asylum. If White employed resurrection men – and there's no evidence one way or the other as to this – why would he take the body of someone so well-connected and closely associated with him?

Was it possible that Hannah was subjected to a post-mortem? This practice was increasing during the eighteenth century, and could be carried out if the patient had a condition that warranted further study. A small number of people did actively request this sort of afterlife. In 1764, for instance, Bristol surgeon Abraham Ludlow wrote up a case, claiming that his patient had known he was dying and:

> That he might be as useful to the world after death as possible, he desired that he might be opened, and, if any thing extraordinary occurred, that it might be published. In order to have this done in an exact manner, his son gave me the liberty of preserving the diseased parts.[29]

An even smaller number of people – in fact, probably just one person – expressed a desire to be included in the anatomical cabinet of a famous anatomist and displayed to an audience. The author Tobias Smollett wrote to John Hunter in 1771 to say: 'You shall receive my poor carcase in a box, after I am dead, to be placed among your rarities.'[30]

In the event, Smollett was not placed among Hunter's rarities, as his wife stepped in and refused to ship his corpse from Italy. But it's an intriguing idea … what if someone, with the agency and capacity to make that decision, actually *wanted* to be in a museum?

If Smollett had made his own pre-death arrangements to have his body shipped to Hunter, would he have taken his place next to Maria van Butchell and Miss Johnson in the end?

And all this brings us back to Hannah. It can't have escaped your notice that Hannah's will specified that three of her close associates remained at Cheetwood Hall for two years after her death. In the accounts of William Hunter and John Sheldon's experiments with embalming, there are references to the body being kept in a box, undisturbed, for a number of years. Were Mary, Esther and Sarah instructed to hold a vigil over Hannah's body at Cheetwood Hall, while the turpentine and oil of lavender did their work?

Of course, that would mean that Hannah not only wanted to be embalmed, but that her family and closest friends knew her wishes and helped to carry them out. And in return, they were handsomely rewarded.

The desire to be dissected and displayed after death is an odd one. Clearly, some people do have this desire, as, in more recent times, the work of Gunther von Hagens and the *Body Worlds* exhibition requires people to 'donate' their body for just this purpose.[31] And Smollett's letter to John Hunter suggests that this might have been a desire that existed in the eighteenth century as well.

Did Hannah want this? Or could there be another reason that she asked Charles White to embalm her body?

Before we consider this possibility, it might be worth taking a closer look at the town in which Hannah and Charles White lived.

11

The pious band

The Manchester I have described so far is a rather genteel Georgian town characterized by ambition and wealth. It's a town where well-to-do doctors practise in King Street and bicker about who should be king, where wealthy spinsters worry about what to give the Duke of Devonshire as a feudal tribute and powerful merchants gather at coffee houses and the Exchange, where the working classes enjoy lectures on chemistry or an art exhibition, or a trip to the Manchester Races. The greatest village in England.

Cottonopolis – the world's first industrial city – seems far away. It would be almost a century after the death of Hannah Beswick before Friedrich Engels would visit Manchester and describe its slums as 'hell on earth', or the Cholera Riots would rip through Angel Meadow.[1] Cottonopolis, a town (and then city) marked by immense inequalities, the nouveau-serfdom of the factory workers, and public health crises, such as cholera epidemics, byssinosis (cotton lung), typhoid, scarlet fever and diphtheria, is a vision of Victorian Manchester. The Georgian Manchester of Hannah Beswick and Dr White seems positively idyllic by comparison. In his book on Angel Meadow, Dean Kirby conjures up a memorable image of pre-industrial Manchester by describing what would become the town's most notorious slum (Engels's 'hell on earth') as a vision of paradise: 'the hillside that formed the steep slope of Angel Street was once a lush grazing pasture [filled with] the sweet melody of skylarks'.[2]

And yet, there was trouble in paradise.

Within a lonely Cott whose tott'ring Wall,
Two rotten Props by just forbad to fall,
Where Wind and Rain an easy Entrance found,

Thro' the wide Chinks that rudely gap'd around,
Lay *Poverty* – her squalid Looks confest
The Piteous Wretch, of Wretches most distrest;
Here the sharp Tooth of biting Want was felt,
Here dire *Disease*, her deepest Dolours dealt,
To prove what Pangs Mortality could bear.

A few loose Straws within the Hovel spread,
Form'd on the Clay-cold Floor her painful Bed,
Whilst baleful Dews distill'd on every Side,
Checking with chilly Damps the Vital Tide.
A Block of Wood, her Pillow, served to raise
Her Head reclin'd, and shew her ghastly Face
With deepest Furroughs plough'd, all wan and pale
As sick'ning Lillies, drooping in the Dale;
Sunk in the Socket was the closing Eye,
The ruddy Cheek had lost each Vermeil Dye,
A lifeless Corse she seem'd, grim Famine's Prey,
Torn immaturely from the World away.

A moving Spectacle – around her press
An infant Brood of Orphans in Distress,
One lifts her languid Arm, and one her Head,
Piercing th'echoing Heav'ns with Cries – for Bread.
Rous'd at the Call, *Compassion* thither came
Led by *Religion*, bright celestial Dame,
Heart-burst she rais'd the Mother from the Ground,
And strove to pour a Balm into the Wound,
With fruitless Pains, her Zeal for want of Art
Serv'd just to ease, but not to cure the Smart.
The helpless Offspring next employ'd her Care,
She fed the hungry, and she cloath'd the bare,
But still that Source of Life from when they sprung,
On whose fond Care, their future Welfare hung
Lay just expiring, the last rising Sigh
Ready to teach us what it is – to die.[3]

This poem appeared on the front page of the *Manchester Mercury* on Tuesday 10 June 1755. Its emotive verses describe the deathbed of a woman who is dying of poverty, starvation and disease, and who 'Compassion' and 'Religion' can only comfort, but not cure.

The poem appeared in the newspaper some sixteen years before Richard Arkwright opened his Cromford Mills, kicking off the industrial revolution for real. (Or, if you prefer the earlier date, some nine years before James Hargreaves invented the Spinning Jenny.) However, although 1755 might not have been a time of 'revolution', it was certainly a time of change.

Enclosure of common land – a practice that likely began in the twelfth century – became normal practice in the eighteenth century. Prior to enclosure, the land of a 'manor' would include some common land, waste or open fields. While these might be under the control of the lord of the manor, they were the spaces that could be used by all manorial tenants. Tenants could take a certain amount of wood from the forests, for instance, or let their pigs into the woods so that they could feed on fallen nuts. Wastelands might include mosses, or bogs, where peat could be obtained for fires or peasants could scratch out some meagre farming. Common lands allowed the possibility of subsistence farming, where manorial tenants could grow enough for their families to survive and, potentially, save enough money to finance tenancies for the next generation.

When common land was enclosed, subsistence farming became harder. Originally, enclosure was carried out by informal agreement between the lord of the manor and his tenants, who were usually financially compensated for their loss of common land. By the eighteenth century, however, an increasing number of Parliamentary Inclosure Acts were being passed to allow individual landlords to enclose the common lands on their manor with parliamentary authority. By the 1750s, when Hannah was living at Cheetwood Hall (possibly with Mary Greame), Parliamentary Inclosure Acts had replaced informal agreement as the main route to enclosure.

As subsistence farming became more difficult, more people switched to agricultural labour as a way of making a living. But being a hired labourer, while it gave you the option of moving from farm to farm looking for the best paid work, was also very difficult. If crops were failing, it might not be possible to find any work at all, or if there were more people looking for work than there was work to do, wages might drop to a lower rate. It was also seasonal work, so you might get four shillings for eleven days' of ploughing after Plough Monday, but you wouldn't see wages like that again until the harvest.[4] At the same time, the price of food (because you're not growing your own) was fluctuating in an inverse proportion to your wages – if the crops failed, you got less work, but the price of bread went up.[5] In the period between 1620 and 1759, there were fifty-nine harvests that were 'deficient' or 'bad', with one eighteenth-century harvest (in 1756) being classed as a 'dearth'.[6] There were food riots in 1756–57, including an incident at Manchester on market day, 7 June 1757, when a group of women and boys were joined by a 'rabble' to attack the potato market, overturn sacks and then plunder the mealhouse.[7] In November 1757, two days of violence at a mealhouse in Manchester saw up to 600 people getting involved, and it resulted in the deaths of one civilian and two of the soldiers who were sent in to quell the mob.[8] By 1760, corn was being imported from overseas to make up the deficiency, a circumstance that would make it even harder to find work as an agricultural labourer and, later on, lead to the passing of the controversial Corn Laws.

If you didn't fancy work as an agricultural labourer, there was always textile production. Until the advent of the industrial revolution – whether you're measuring that by the Spinning Jenny or the Water Frame – textile production was done in the home, on spinning wheels and handlooms. Manchester was a town long associated with textiles. 'Manchester Cottons' were an Elizabethan, not a Victorian, creation, as weavers in the town had developed a method of raising ('cottoning') the nap of a woollen cloth to create a distinctive fabric as early as 1551.[9] Early modern merchants operated from the streets close to the Collegiate Church, including Cateaton Street, Smithy Door and The Shambles. One exporter of Manchester Cottons was Nicholas Mosley, who was so successful a clothier, he was able to buy the lordship of the manor of Manchester in 1596 for £3,500. We've met (slightly distant) relatives of his in previous chapters: Lady Ann Bland's father, Oswald Mosley, was the third cousin once removed of Nicholas Mosley's great-grandson Edward.

But, of course, not everyone involved in Manchester Cottons or the growing fustian trade was a Nicholas Mosley. Most were people weaving and spinning at home. At first, the successful world of Manchester textiles operated on a commercial system that saw merchants trading in yarn or buying woven material to finish and then market for a profit. However, by the eighteenth century, a system known as 'putting out' had become the dominant mode of business. Essentially, this was outsourcing. A clothier would buy raw materials and pay workers to complete each step of the fabric's production. Michael Nevell has suggested that this system came into play in Manchester as early as the 1680s.[10]

The seventeenth- and early eighteenth-century 'putting out' system was lucrative for merchants and clothiers. For instance, Nevell gives the example of Joseph Jolly, who died in 1753, leaving over £430 of stock in his warehouse, £550 of stock in his weigh-house, and records of thirteen yarn winders and forty-two weavers with whom he'd been working.[11] While that might have been good news for Jolly, the payments made to yarn winders and weavers were becoming more and more precarious as time went on. This was partly due to the fluctuating price of both raw materials and finished goods, as commercial markets are never stable. It was also partly due to increased regulation and taxation on cotton goods, in various attempts to protect the 'homegrown' wool trade. The Manchester Act 1736 prohibited the manufacture of all-cotton cloths in Britain, and placed a tax of 3d. per yard on cotton mix fabrics such as fustian. The reduced profits for the clothiers would, of course, mean lower wages for the weavers.

Working in the textile trade, particularly if you could get work as a weaver, was a decidedly better option in early eighteenth-century Manchester than working as an agricultural labourer, but the work was generally piecework. And the problem with it being a better option was that there was more competition for work, as increasing numbers of people gave up on agricultural labour and moved to the town in search of more secure work, either making fabric, finishing fabrics or working in the warehouses and weigh-houses that were required for the trade.

* * *

In the poem that appeared in the *Manchester Mercury* in 1755, the dying mother is a victim of poverty and famine, both of which could have been the result of the changing economy of the town and its rural neighbours. However, she's also a victim of disease, and so it's worth looking at what this might have meant in the first half of the eighteenth century.

First of all, smallpox was endemic in Manchester at this time, and it was the cause of somewhere between 10 and 20 per cent of deaths. The fact that it was endemic meant that it was persistently present in the region, and evidence shows that smallpox deaths were most common in children, suggesting that most people who made it to adulthood had already survived the disease and acquired immunity.[12] Influenza and typhus epidemics hit periodically as well, replacing plague, which had caused devastation in the previous century. And then there was putrid fever, hysteric fever, nervous fever, gangrene, bloody flux, French pox, rising of the lights and St Anthony's Fire to contend with.[13]

These illnesses were not discriminatory. Hannah Beswick saw the deaths of four monarchs during her lifetime. The first, Mary II, who died when Hannah was still a baby, died of smallpox. Mary's husband and co-monarch William III died shortly afterwards from pneumonia caused by a broken collarbone. Queen Anne survived smallpox, but it killed three of her children. Only George I managed to avoid fatal illness, eventually succumbing to a stroke.

If even monarchs could not survive smallpox and pneumonia, what hope did a poor starving woman in a hovel have?

The developments in medical education I talked about in previous chapters offered some solace to the upper classes. The anatomist William Hunter, for instance, would go on to become the physician to Queen Charlotte, the wife of George III. And before that, Hans Sloane, later president of the College of Physicians, would serve as first physician to George II. Other physicians and surgeons, like Manchester's Charles White, might not rise to such lofty positions, but they would certainly gain the status to command high fees from their wealthy patients. These doctors even pioneered techniques for inoculation against smallpox, prior to the development of a vaccination in 1796, which involved administering small amounts of the virus into open wounds. Quite a lot of people inoculated in this way survived (though not all), and it became a desirable treatment.

Most people couldn't afford to pay a doctor like Charles White. For people a little lower on the social hierarchy, there were other medical practitioners available, such as bone-setters, barbers, apothecaries and herbalists. There was also a wide range of patent medicines available, such as Dr James's Fever Powders, which allegedly cured a man who simultaneously suffered an outbreak of smallpox *and* rabies, and which could be bought at the New Tea Warehouse, next door to the Long-Room in Manchester.[14] Or Warham's Apoplectick Snuff, which prevented 'infections, such as Small-Pox', and cost 6d. a box or 1s. per ounce, and Dr Lower's Purging Paste, a treatment against both worms and scurvy at 1s. a box (also available from the New Tea Warehouse in Manchester).[15]

But what of the people who couldn't even afford a shilling for Dr Lower's Purging Paste? What became of them?

The concept of 'poor relief' dates back to the late Middle Ages, but it became something more systematic in the Elizabethan period. In the sixteenth century, this took the form of charity, such as the distribution of food and clothing, at a parish level. The Act of Relief for the Poor 1597 and then the Poor Relief Act 1601 codified this. Mostly, these early acts of poor relief weren't intended as a progressive 'welfare system', but rather a way of dealing with vagabonds, vagrants and beggars. Alms (food and clothing given to the poor) would be distributed to the needy by the parish, so anyone begging for money or refusing to seek work would be sanctioned. Sanctions included, in 1547, two years' servitude and branding with the letter 'V', and, in 1572, being 'bored through the ear'.

Almhouses – again a medieval creation – continued to operate throughout the early modern period as places to house those who were unable to work or provide for themselves, such as widows, orphans, older people and physically disabled people. Although these institutions were often called 'hospitals', they weren't set up to care for the sick, but rather to offer subsidized accommodation for the 'deserving poor'. Many almshouses had chapels, and so, with the Abolition of Chantries Acts 1545 and 1547, they gave way to poorhouses (accommodation) and workhouses (employment). The Poor Relief Act of 1601 set out the differing arrangements for such institutions: the 'impotent poor' (those who couldn't work due to age or disability) would go to the poorhouse; those of 'sufficient ability' would go to the workhouse; and the 'idle poor' would go to a house of correction.

The administrative unit for poor relief was the parish, meaning that the parish now had the responsibility of providing poor relief for anyone 'impotent', 'of sufficient ability' or 'idle' who needed it within the area around the parish church. They were also responsible for raising the requisite funds to provide this relief through a 'poor rate' collected from local property owners. The Act would continue to be in force through the eighteenth century, when it was added to by the provision of the Poor Relief or Work House Test Act 1722, which stated that anyone wanting to claim poor relief had to undertake a set amount of work in the workhouse before receiving any help.[16]

And none of this would treat your scurvy or reset a broken bone. If you contracted a fever or a contagious disease in the poorhouse, you would simply just pass it on to everyone else and pray for your survival.

The poem in the *Manchester Mercury* in 1755 reveals the limitations of charity and almsgiving. As the poor woman lies dying, her children crying out for bread, Compassion (personified) immediately hears her call. Compassion is accompanied by Religion, of course, as these are imagined as the two main reasons for giving charity.

But Compassion and Religion are powerless to help, not through want of kindness, but through 'want of art'. Compassion and Religion just aren't qualified to deal with the effects of disease and starvation. They can ease the pain but never cure it.

However, the poem doesn't end there. Compassion, realizing her limits, puts out a call for help. She assembles 'a goodly Train' who unite to save the poor woman, and others like her. Compassion's 'Train' will create something new – something not seen before in the town:

> Here the foul Gangrene ranckling to the Bone,
> Shall stop its putrid Course – the tort'ring Stone
> Shall quit its Lodgment, yielding to the Knife,
> Nor longer Poison every Sweet of Life.
> The God of Health, with rosy-colour'd Plume,
> Shall visit daily each salubrious Room,
> And as he passes every Heart shall swell,
> With Gratitude too strong for Tongue to tell –
> She said and straight issued forth the pious Band,
> And *an Infirmary* rose to bless the Land.[17]

You see, this poem wasn't actually a sentimental lament about the cruelties of poverty. It was a triumphant hymn to the Manchester Infirmary, founded three years earlier in the centre of town by, among others, Dr Charles White.

* * *

An infirmary was a voluntary hospital, set up as an independent institution funded through donations and subscriptions by wealthy benefactors. Treatment was provided by 'honorary' (i.e. voluntary) physicians and surgeons, and management was provided by a committee of governors. The ancestor of the infirmary is St Bartholemew's Hospital (also known as Barts) in London, which began as a medieval almshouse in the twelfth century. St Mary Bethlehem (also known as Bedlam) had similar roots, but while Bedlam developed into an institution that would house – or incarcerate – people with mental and neurological health conditions, Barts transformed into a poorhouse with a focus on cutting-edge general medicine. When Barts was refounded by Henry VIII and given to the Corporation of London after the dissolution of the monasteries, its first superintendent was the king's own surgeon and physician, Thomas Vicary, who was also a leading anatomist. And then, in the seventeenth century, William Harvey conducted his groundbreaking research into the circulatory system at the hospital.

In the eighteenth century, with populations starting to rise in urban areas of the country, other places started to follow the example of Barts. In 1729, Edinburgh got its Hospital for the Sick Poor (later the Royal Infirmary of Edinburgh), and, in 1735, Bristol Infirmary was founded. By the early 1750s, when facing a very rapidly growing population and increasing urban poverty and disease, Manchester decided to follow suit.

The plan for the infirmary was set in motion in 1751, when a group of men – George Floyd, esq., John Lees, Miles Bower and Joseph Bancroft – met at a coffeehouse and came up with a proposal for raising donations and subscriptions for the new hospital. A subscription would differ from a donation, as it would bestow the right to refer potential patients to the infirmary. The *Manchester Mercury*, a newspaper founded by the staunch Tory Joseph Harrop, was keen to point out that subscribing to the infirmary would actually help landowners to avoid paying out too much poor relief or alms, as if they were approached by someone seeking aid due to 'infirmity', they could just refer them to the infirmary and not feel they had to offer financial support.

However, it's not fair to assume those motivations in all the men involved in founding the infirmary, as most of them worked for free to offer healthcare to poorer residents of the town. This was initially somewhat limited, as the first premises they secured was a house on Garden Street, near Withy Grove, which could only accommodate twelve patients. By then though, they had secured the support of Charles White, who was twenty-four years old and fresh from his training under William Hunter in London, and also his father Thomas, who was appointed Surgeon Extraordinary to the infirmary when it opened in 1752.[18]

Richard Edward Hall was also a Surgeon Extraordinary at the foundation of the hospital, and his son Edward was one of the surgeons, along with Charles White and James Burchall (who would later be replaced by Hall's other son Richard). The infirmary's original physicians were Peter Mainwaring, Samuel Kay and James Walker. This, according to the *Manchester Mercury*, was Compassion's 'goodly train', the 'pious band'.

Within a year, the infirmary had to expand, taking on the neighbouring house on Garden Street in order to do so, and by 1755 it needed its own purpose-built location. A new infirmary was constructed on land then known as the Daub-Holes (because it was the site of clay used for the daub in wattle-and-daub houses), which was directly opposite the house where Ashton Lever would display his natural history cabinet eleven years later. This area of the town is probably better known by its current name: Piccadilly Gardens.

There is so much more that could be said about the development of the Manchester Infirmary (now Manchester Royal Infirmary, or MRI). It was pioneering in its early inclusion of a set of baths, open to both the public and trustees, and for integrating a dispensary into the hospital itself. However, it also faced controversy later in the eighteenth century, when Charles White, his son Thomas and the Halls fell out with the governing committee about plans to expand the number of patients who could be taken in, and the number of 'home patients' that could be treated. This was, in part, a political dispute with the Tories (the Whites and the Halls) facing off against a largely Whig-supporting committee, but it was also a question of public health versus individual medical practice, and nepotism versus the inclusion of wider expertise. In the end, the Whites and the Halls lost the support of the committee, and they left the infirmary to found a new institution, the Lying-In Charity, which would open the doors of its maternity hospital (now St Mary's) in 1790.[19]

But this isn't really the story of the Manchester Infirmary, it's the story of Hannah Beswick. And, while a lot of things in her story have to rely on conjecture, there is one fact that I can be sure of: Hannah was an early, and generous, supporter of the new hospital.

In 1752, Hannah donated £40 to the new infirmary. While this might not seem a lot at first glance, Hannah's donation was the third highest received at this point, beaten only by the Earl of Warrington (who gave £42) and Sir Ralph Assheton, baronet (who gave £50). In 1754, the Earl of Warrington upped his donation to £68 5s., and by then Sir Thomas Grey Egerton, baronet, had donated £52, and Sir Oswald Mosley, baronet, had chipped in £50. I mention this by way of context for Hannah's £40, as she contributed a similar amount to earls, knights and baronets.

By 1754, lots of the people we have met in the story so far had either given a donation or paid for a subscription to the infirmary. Thomas Gorton, the Byroms and Ashton Lever were among the subscribers, and money had also been raised at collections in the Collegiate Church, St Ann's Church and the Cross Street Chapel. Over 2,000 patients had been treated in the hospital by this point.

When Hannah died in 1758, she left money to the infirmary, adding a codicil to her will with the instruction that £100 was to be given to the Trustees of the 'Publick Infirmary' so it could be 'applyed towards carrying on the charitable designs of that society'. This isn't a particularly large bequest for someone with Hannah's wealth – in the inventory of her will from 1761, we can see that she had over £500 in cash in her house when she died – but I think it's significant that Hannah added this legacy to the earlier donation she made.

I don't think Hannah was donating to ensure the right to refer alms-seekers to the infirmary and so avoid having to deal with them herself, as the *Manchester Mercury* advised. Had she been looking to do this, she would have bought a subscription rather than making a 'benefaction'. On the other hand, I don't think we can assume Hannah was particularly interested in the care of the poor, outside a general awareness that a wealthy person should do something for charity.

What's interesting is that Hannah is an early donor, and that her name appears alongside the fashionable elite of the town. When the infirmary was seeking donations to its cause in 1752, the founders contacted the great and the good *directly* to solicit their donations. The much wider list of 1754 shows that the cause had become a bit trendy (everyone who was anyone had a subscription to the infirmary), but the donors in 1752 were a smaller group, most likely known – at least by reputation – to the 'pious band'. Someone, whether it was Charles White or one of the merchants, like Joseph Bancroft, who came up with the original infirmary proposal, knew Hannah well enough to ask her for money. And she trusted them enough to give it. It's important to remember that there was no real precedent, outside of Bristol and Edinburgh, for the public infirmary planned in Manchester, and so any donations would have to be given on faith.

Who did Hannah have faith in? George Floyd, John Lees, Miles Bower and Joseph Bancroft? Or the man to whom she would, six years later, entrust not only the execution of her last will and testament, but also the handling of her mortal remains?

12

Four hundred pounds

When Hannah Beswick died, she left £400 to cover the expense of her funeral. As we saw in earlier chapters, this has been a source of suspicion in later years, with some people going so far as to suggest Charles White embalmed Hannah's body and put it in his museum so that he could pocket the money for himself. Other people have suggested that Hannah's family – who were to get any surplus left from the money – skimped on the funeral in order to keep more of the cash.

The question that has never really been asked is, what did Hannah expect to get for that £400? What sort of funeral would she have expected for the money?

When Hannah's body was finally buried in Harpurhey Cemetery in 1868, Robert Dukinfield Darbishire, acting on behalf of the Commissioners of the Natural History Society, employed a firm of undertakers to oversee the arrangements, Satterfield and Company, who were based at St Ann's Square. In a nicely respectful touch, Darbishire had employed one of the most prestigious undertakers in the city.

Satterfield's were established in 1775, as linen drapers rather than undertakers, and, by 1868, their premises at 9–17 St Ann's Square were a showroom for the clothing lines, fabrics, hosiery and millinery that they stocked. The 'private house' door at No. 13 was for funerals and 'mourning orders', and this had different opening hours to the rest of the business.

Ten years before Hannah's body was buried, Satterfield's had attended to the funeral of the Countess of Wilton, who died in 1858 of typhoid fever and congestion of the lungs. The undertakers arranged the transportation of the countess's body from Melton Mowbray (where she died) to Heaton Park in Prestwich, near Manchester (the family seat of the Wiltons). Once at Heaton Park, the body was 'deposited in one of the state bedchambers, where it remained until the funeral'. The countess's funeral cortège included two mutes 'carrying escutcheons', eight underbearers, funeral feathers and a hearse drawn by six horses. This was followed by nine mourning coaches, family carriages and other private carriages. The funeral procession entered the church to Handel's 'Dead March' from *Saul*, played on the organ. And the 'deceased countess was enclosed in three coffins, the outer one of which was covered with purple silk velvet'.[1]

This was far from the only high-profile funeral Satterfield's arranged. The following year, they handled the mortal remains of James Pownall, esq., J. P., arranging a funeral cortège of two mutes, a hearse drawn by four horses, six mourning coaches and private carriages. After the funeral, James Pownall's body was deposited in a brick vault, and 'many hundreds of workpeople and neighbours visited the grave, and took a final look at the coffin it contained'. Reports of this funeral noted that the 'funeral was conducted by Messrs Satterfield and Sons, the eminent undertakers of St Ann's Square, Manchester, and all the arrangements were efficiently superintended by Mr Oliver, of their establishment'.[2]

Three years later, 'the solemn rite of burial was paid to the mortal remains of the late Mr John Robinson Kay', a wealthy Bury businessman and director of the East Lancashire Railway. Again, Satterfield's handled the arrangements for this, including placing the body in 'three coffins (half a ton in weight the whole) the inner one being of oak, next to which was one of lead, and the outer one a beautiful and massive coffin of oak, French polished, with fine brass mountings'. The triple-coffin was brought in a 'hearse was drawn by four horses, dark as the raven's plume, and each of the seven mourning coaches was drawn by two black horses'. On arrival at the Wesleyan chapel, where the funeral was to take place:

> The coffin had been placed on a bier and covered with a handsome velvet pall, three beautiful wreaths of immortelles, &c., were placed thereon,

> after which the mourners, &c., proceeded into the building (the railway employees having filed along either side of the pathway), while the soul-thrilling strains of the 'Dead March' in Saul came in subdued tones from the organ.[3]

Now, we know that this wasn't quite the style of funeral Satterfield's arranged for Hannah. Darbishire asked them to refrain from the expense of a single oak coffin, let alone three coffins that weighed half a ton in total. However, it's clear from the comments that appeared after the burial of her body that some people believed that this sort of pomp was what Hannah had in mind when she left £400 to cover funeral expenses. The money she specified in her will was to cover the cost of undertakers, mutes, hearses, an organist playing the 'Dead March', and mourning coaches for her family. Obviously, none of that happened, so her final wishes must have been ignored by her family, who took the money and gave her body to Charles White.

The thing is, Hannah died over a century before her burial. And a lot can change in a century.

* * *

Prior to the eighteenth century, funerals in England were, primarily, a religious matter. Religious rites were performed, and then the body was interred (in the ground, in a crypt or in a vault, depending on the family practice). Cremation, while it was practised in pre-Christian Britain – think about the funeral pyre in *Beowulf*, for instance – was not an accepted means for disposing of mortal remains in medieval and early modern England. Christian doctrine taught that the dead would be 'resurrected' into Heaven on the Day of Judgement, and so the disintegration of the corpse through burning would prevent this from happening. Burial, then, was preferred, and by the early modern period this generally meant being placed in a box and buried in a churchyard.

Of course, the prohibition on cremation meant that every single person who died had to be buried, apart from those people who had committed crimes or sins that meant their bodies were 'unworthy' of burial, and so they were gibbeted, displayed, dismembered or otherwise destroyed after death. The population of early modern England was undoubtedly far smaller than the present day, but still, that's a lot of bodies to bury. In times of crisis, like an outbreak of plague, it was a lot of bodies that had to be buried in a short space of time, and so mass graves ('plague pits') might be used. Interred bodies were often stacked on top of one another in graves, with the most recent burial being really quite close to the surface. In addition to this, as churchyards were necessarily alongside churches, they were subject to movement. Churches close and are rebuilt elsewhere; populations of towns change, requiring church land to be repurposed. In the medieval and early modern period, the disinterment of bodies as a result of overcrowding or relocation of churchyards was not uncommon. And neither was accidental disinterment, as old graves were easily disturbed when a new burial was occurring. The idea of 'six feet under' applies only to the first coffin placed in a grave, with that depth supposedly allowing two further coffins to be placed on top before the grave is full. It's clear that, in some churchyards and cemeteries, attempts were made to go beyond that by starting a little deeper to fit more than three coffins in.

So, whose help did you need if you were arranging an early modern funeral? Let's think about the funeral of Hannah's mother in 1695, for instance. Who would that have involved?

The first person, of course, would be the parish priest. Hannah's mother was buried at the Collegiate Church, so the priest there would have agreed the burial and registered the death. Next, there would be a gravedigger, employed by the church. At smaller, rural churches, gravediggers might be employed on a 'freelance' basis, working in other professions as their 'day job' and digging graves at night for extra income. But at larger churches – like Manchester's Collegiate Church – there would be a sexton or team of sextons, who were employed to maintain the church building and its churchyard, ring the bells and dig the graves. The gravediggers in *Hamlet* are perhaps the most famous depiction of the profession in this period, and they refer to themselves as 'sextons'.

Hannah's mother would have been placed in a coffin, but it's unlikely to have been an ostentatious triple coffin as we saw in the nineteenth-century funerals directed by Satterfield's. It would have been a wooden coffin, likely made of elm or perhaps oak, and possibly lined with some sort of fabric, which would have been purchased from a coffin-maker. Poorer people at the time were often buried without a coffin, just wrapped in a shroud, but the Beswick family would have been able to meet the expense of a coffin-maker. Coffin-makers in the late seventeenth century were, as you would imagine, carpenters, many of whom were furniture makers by trade – a coffin is not so different to a cabinet, after all. However, upholsterers and metalworkers were also involved in coffin-making, and stonemasons were employed to carve headstones.

Before being placed in the coffin, a body would have to be wrapped in a shroud, and this would need to be purchased from someone working with textiles. Linen shrouds were commonly used in the seventeenth century, partly due to availability and partly due to religious sensibilities. In the Christian tradition, linen shrouds were desirable, as Jesus was wrapped in linen. This wasn't good for the local woollen industry though, so the Wool Act of 1667, which placed various restrictions on the use of linen, mandated that bodies must be buried in woollen shrouds. The only exception made was for plague victims, because of the belief that wool remained infected by plague. In 1677, the Wool Act was strengthened, imposing a fine of £5 on any burial using other fabrics.

Prior to being wrapped in the shroud, the body would be laid out, washed and dressed with sweet-smelling herbs like rosemary and bay to mask decay. While this sounds quite charming, the 'laying out' of a corpse would also include emptying the bowels and plugging the orifices. Before the seventeenth century, this task generally fell to the family of the deceased, but it later became a job to be arranged by the coffin-maker, who would 'outsource' the task to local women.[4] Aristocratic and royal corpses might receive further treatment, being 'embalmed' or chemically preserved to prevent putrefaction. One of the main reasons for this is that high-profile funerals (for instance, for the monarch) might not take place immediately after death. If there were questions around succession or inheritance, or if heirs were overseas at the time of death, the funeral might have to be delayed, and the body was at risk of decomposition in the meantime. Not pleasant for the bereaved relatives, but also not good for the soul of the deceased who might have to approach the Day of Judgement as a mouldering corpse. The tradition of keeping royal bodies 'lying in state', in which the body of a monarch or head of state is placed in a state building in order to allow the public to pay their respects, dates back to the seventeenth century and, for the sake of public decency, does require the body to have undergone some degree of preservation to mask the signs of decay from the grieving populace.[5]

The methods employed for this type of post-mortem preservation included the removal of internal organs, which were then buried separately to the body, washing internal cavities with aromatic fluids, treating the outside of the body with spices, and then wrapping the corpse tightly in waxed fabric with sealed seams to ensure it was as airtight as possible.[6] From the Middle Ages onwards, a more dramatic technique had to be employed for monarchs who died overseas, as the body would have to stay 'preserved' for the long journey to transport it to the site of burial.

The 'Mos Teutonicus' (or 'German custom') was developed during the time of the Holy Roman Empire, after Charlemagne outlawed the practice of cremation, arguing that destroying someone's bones was equivalent to destroying their soul. This practice was used to preserve the bones of a dead person for transportation, in the event that there was no chance of preventing decomposition of the flesh. The corpse would be dismembered, with the heart and intestines removed. Body parts were then boiled in milk, wine or vinegar to remove the flesh from the bones. The flesh and internal organs could then either be buried 'in situ' or salted, like meat, for preservation. The skeleton was sprinkled with perfume and shipped to the place of burial. This practice died out in the fifteenth century; however, it was replaced with other methods of preserving and storing a royal body, which continued into the Georgian period.

For someone like Hannah's mother, versions of the 'Mos Teutonicus' were unnecessary, and the aristocratic method of embalming was not very likely. As an upper-middle-class, almost gentry, woman, it is most likely that her body was carefully washed and dressed by local lower-class women employed by either the church or the coffin-maker, and then wrapped in a woollen shroud (unless her family decided to pay the fine for using linen). Her family were wealthy enough for a headstone to be erected, or an existing family stone to be amended, and she would have been buried in a wooden coffin prepared for her, probably with a tin or other metal plate attached to it bearing her name.

The cost to the family would have included money to the priest, the sextons and other church personnel, the fee to the coffin-maker for coffin, coffin furniture and preparation of the body, the cost of providing funeral food for mourners, and, perhaps, clothing for the family to wear to the funeral itself. Mourning attire was not such big business as it would become in the nineteenth century, when Manchester had Bateman's Mourning Warehouse on Oldham Street, which could provide complete outfits 'for every grade in mourning' and copy any new style from London and Paris 'at economical prices' (just send a telegram to 'Mourning, Manchester' or telephone No. 615).[7] When Hannah's mother died in 1695, it was common to provide gloves and, perhaps, new hats and accessories, but nothing elaborate enough to warrant a 'Mourning Warehouse'. Adding all this up, this average cost of a gentry funeral at this time was around £50.[8]

Between her mother's death and Hannah's own, some things had started to change in the practice of arranging funerals. The first half of the eighteenth century saw what has been described as the 'professionalisation of death'.[9] Tradespeople who made coffins – usually furniture-makers or upholsterers – began to offer wider services. As these artisans would have connections with other tradespeople, like drapers, cloth manufacturers and metalworkers, as part of their everyday business, they were perfectly placed to coordinate the different services required for a burial. For a fee, they could handle every undertaking for the bereaved family.

The rise of the entrepreneurial undertaker in the early eighteenth century had an impact on funeral practices and customs. At this point in time, there was a marked difference between the funerals of different classes of people. A poor person's funeral would use the reusable 'parish coffin' to transport the shrouded body to the churchyard, while the aristocracy could purchase single-use coffins made of oak and with brass decoration and fabric upholstery that would be buried in the ground with the body. The middle classes might not have been able to afford the pomp and circumstance of an aristocratic funeral, but they would certainly aspire to that over the more anonymous treatment of the pauper's body.

Professional undertakers could use their trade contacts to provide funeral services for middle-class people that incorporated some of the panache of an upper-class burial. They could provide a coffin with a tin nameplate, if brass was out of budget. And they could ensure the coffin was lined with flannel or bran (useful for absorbing the liquids of a putrefying corpse) to mimic the use of crêpe and silk in more expensive affairs.[10] As a result, the use of a coffin, complete with decoration and lining, became commonplace, even in the funerals of the less well off.

As well as embalming, aristocratic and royal funerals had long made use of double- or triple-shelled coffins, with both wooden and lead cases, presumably another necessary precaution against a delayed burial. These 'coffin-within-a-coffin' arrangements became a 'metropolitan fashion' in the eighteenth century, and provincial undertakers sought to copy the style for their customers.[11] A coffin of this sort required both a carpenter and a plumber (i.e. a lead worker), and so an undertaker would coordinate these contractors on behalf of their customers.

In turn, these changing practices also affected perceptions and beliefs about death itself. As coffins ceased to be practical wooden boxes used to contain a shrouded body and came to be decorated and lined receptacles in which the deceased would repose until Judgement Day, the idea of death as sleep became more prominent. Lining a coffin with yards of white crêpe transformed it from a box into a bed, and eighteenth-century undertakers enhanced this effect by offering the inclusion of a pillow under the corpse's head or a sheet to pull over the body.[12]

As coffins became more elaborate affairs, they required different modes of transportation. The funerals of the aristocracy had long involved the use of hearses. Originally, the word 'hearse' referred to a wooden or metal frame placed over a coffin on its bier (the stand on which a coffin is placed to either lie in state or await transportation to a burial site) to support the pall (the decorated cloth placed over the coffin). The word then came to refer to any construction into which a coffin was placed, before acquiring its more specific seventeenth-century meaning of a *vehicle* into which a coffin was placed for transportation. A hearse could be – and often was – a handcart, but for wealthier families it would be a horse-drawn vehicle.

Undertakers, originally, would not have had their own hearses. At a time when even the wealthiest families might not own a private carriage, a vehicle of this sort (plus the horses and stables it would require) was beyond the reach of even the most entrepreneurial undertaker. However, they could be hired in for the occasion. In his exploration of early undertaking practice in the West Country, Daniel O'Brien has identified a number of eighteenth-century establishments that offered hearses for hire, including a linen draper and undertaker in Chippenham, who would hire his vehicle for use in 'any part of England', and several public houses and hotels, like The Bear in Bath, who kept and hired out hearses.[13]

In 1750s Manchester, maltster Joseph Barret got in on the hearse-hiring business, advertising a mourning coach and hearse 'at the most reasonable' rates, on enquiry at his premises opposite the Saracen's Head or at the Swan With Two Necks on Market-street-lane.[14] Other establishments were also capitalizing on the 'professionalisation of death' and the changes to funeral fashions this entailed. For example, in 1753, just five years before Hannah's death, the premises of John Berry, grocer, in Manchester (also known as the New Tea Warehouse, stockists of Dr James's Fever Powders and Dr Lower's Purging Paste) were advertising 'flamboys' (torches) for 'funeral processions', which had 'just arrived from London'.[15] And when James Lowe and Ralph Bate purchased a draper's shop and stock in trade from the Byrom family in 1762, they quickly advertised 'stripped silks' that were 'now selling very cheap' and a 'large assortment of black and white silks for funerals always ready'.[16]

The options – and the expectations – for Hannah's funeral in 1758 were far beyond those that were the norm when her mother died some sixty-three years earlier. Her family could have employed an undertaker, bought a triple-shelled coffin lined with lead for decency and decorated with brass handles and plate, hired a hearse from the Saracen's Head, bought flamboys from the New Tea Warehouse, and covered everything with silks and crêpe. They were even rich enough to afford the fine for a linen shroud, if that's what she would've wanted.

The problem is, even with all of this, including a £5 fine under the Wool Act, the funeral expenses wouldn't have come close to reaching £400. In fact, there is evidence that funerals actually got cheaper in the eighteenth century, precisely as a result of the newly competitive market in mourning accoutrements that were 'selling cheap'.[17]

* * *

It's possible I was a bit hasty in claiming that the corpse of Hannah's mother would have been laid out and washed by lower-class women employed by the coffin-maker or church. There were other options for preparing a body for burial, and the Beswicks were a wealthy enough family to perhaps take advantage of some of these.

Even if a funeral didn't need to be delayed, and the body didn't need to lie in state, there were other reasons why a corpse might need to be preserved before burial. The first was a practical one. As I've said, accidental and deliberate exhumations were just a fact of early modern churchyards, with grim reports of gravediggers sticking shovels through old corpses as they opened up new graves. Ideally, if your body was going to be disinterred and revealed at a later date, you'd want it to look its best.

This relates to the second reason why post-mortem preservation was considered important for some people: the Christian idea of Judgement Day, which would see earthly remains translated into heavenly body. Some eighteenth-century clergy were keen to point out that this was not to be taken literally. The 'earthly remains' that would be resurrected were souls, not actual corpses. For instance, in a 1755 Puritan sermon entitled *A Serious Persuasive to Prepare for Death*, the Reverend Thomas Doolittle described death as:

> The destroying and demolishing of the Body of Man, that famous and curious Fabrick, and a bringing it into Dust and Putrefaction, (Psalm 40:3). It turns a living Body into a dead Carcass, a lifeless Lump of Clay; and causeth it to become Meat for Worms to feed on, (Job 18:26).[18]

Nevertheless, the association of the 'uncorrupted corpse' with the heavenly soul was a long-standing one. From the Middle Ages onwards, the bodies of saints were associated with a divine lack of decomposition, setting a pretty high standard for the 'uncorrupted corpse'. It's no wonder some people felt they had to turn to more cosmetic means to achieve this.

Embalming was the obvious way to ensure a corpse retained a more pleasing appearance, either for Judgement Day or for the day when a sexton stuck a spade through your rotted coffin, and in the late seventeenth and early eighteenth centuries this started to become a standard funerary custom for the middle classes, as it had been for the upper classes. In 1727, a wealthy linen draper called Francis Bancroft laid out instructions for his mortal remains in his will: 'My Body I desire may be embalmed within six Days after my Death, and my Entrails to be put in a Leaden Box, and included in my Coffin, or placed in my Vault next the same, as shall be most convenient.'[19] The 'Leaden Box' Bancroft specifies is a viscera box, in which the internal organs were placed when a body was embalmed for a funeral. It would either be buried with the body in its coffin or placed in a special niche in a vault or tomb. Significantly, Bancroft's will of 1727 attaches a price limit to his funeral, stating that it must not cost more than £200. This amount is substantially higher than the cost of a coffin, hearse and mourning attire, suggesting that the embalming itself would be one of the most expensive parts of the procedure.

Bancroft – a member of the middle classes, though a wealthy one – required that his viscera box be placed in or near his coffin. The upper classes, however, made different uses of viscera boxes, often keeping them in a different location to the buried corpse. When William, Duke of Gloucester, the son of Princess (later Queen) Anne, died in 1700, his body was disembowelled and embalmed before burial. His entrails were placed in a leaden box, which was taken to Westminster Abbey and placed in the Stuart vault, along with the entrails of several other members of the royal family.[20]

What had been a royal and aristocratic practice born of necessity became a romanticized and sentimental aspiration of the lower nobility and gentry. The idea of keeping organs – or one organ, in particular – separate from the buried corpse became a romantic ideal. The heart, the most symbolic of all the entrails, would be removed on embalming and preserved separately, as an emblem of the deceased's virtuousness in life, or of the bereaved's enduring love for them. Sir William Temple, who died in 1699, was buried at Westminster Abbey, but his heart was placed in a silver box and buried in his garden. James Radclyffe, Earl of Derwentshire, who was executed in 1716 for his part in the '15, had his heart enclosed in a casket and sent to some nuns. Sir Nicholas Cripe, who died in 1739, had his heart placed in an urn, which would be displayed at St Paul's in Hammersmith.[21]

Such practices ceased to be about funeral arrangements and embalming as such, and started to be about the most intense memento mori one could hope to have. The following century, as Percy Shelley's body was cremated in a makeshift pyre on the beach near Viareggio, his friend Leigh Hunt reached into the flames and grabbed the poet's calcified heart. Shelley's widow Mary kept this preserved organ for the rest of her life, although recent studies have suggested it was probably actually his liver.

Romantics aside, the idea of keeping viscera separately from the body grows out of the practice of embalming. As I've said, the methods of embalming used by the early modern aristocracy involved removing internal organs and then applying preservative fluids to the bodily cavities. There was no method of preserving the organs themselves, unless they were salted (as in the case of medieval monarchs who were treated to the 'Mos Teutonicus'). Entrails were the byproduct of preserving the body, not something that needed to be kept 'uncorrupted' in themselves. Presumably, this was partly because it's very hard to imagine the more abject organs, such as the intestines and bowels, as being 'uncorrupt' if you've just had to empty their contents. But it was also an issue of practicality – there was no way of preserving soft organs that really worked. The caskets and silver boxes and urns that enclosed the viscera of the great and the good looked very decorous from the outside, but if you opened them up, you'd find something that resembled the consistency of tinned salmon.

Embalming became an accepted practice in middle-class and gentry funerals in the early eighteenth century. The question was, who would you get to carry out the work?

* * *

In modern-day funerals, embalming is something we expect undertakers to undertake, with the assistance of morticians, who will not only delay the signs of decay but also employ 'the services of the toilet' to render the corpse as lifelike as possible, in case it is to be viewed prior to burial or cremation.

When undertaking emerged as a profession in the early eighteenth century, it's no surprise to find some entrepreneurs offering embalming as part of their package of services. Apothecaries had offered the treatment of corpses as a service for some time, and so the undertakers took over as a 'trade' version of this. This was not looked on favourably by everyone. Thomas Greenhill, writing in 1705, likened undertakers to 'Quacks', stating that it was a shame that society had allowed itself 'to suffer a sort of Men call'd *Undertakers*, to monopolize the several Trades of *Glovers*, *Milliners*, *Drapers*, *Wax-Chandlers*, *Coffin-Makers*, *Herald-Painters*, *Surgeons*, *Apothecaries*, and the like'.[22] Other sources reveal an equal distrust of undertakers, as their role in the commercialization of death was seen as distasteful, dishonest and downright ghoulish.

In his compendium of London trades, written in 1747, R. Campbell gave this assessment of the undertaking trade:

> Their Business is to watch Death, and to furnish out the Funeral Solemnity, with as much Pomp and feigned Sorrow, as the Heirs or Successor of the Deceased chuse to purchase: They are a hard-hearted Generation, and require more Money than Brains to conduct their business: I know of no one Qualification peculiarly necessary to them, except it is a steady, demure and melancholy Countenance at Command; I do not know that they take Apprentices in their Capacity as Undertakers, for they are generally Carpenters, or Herald-Painters besides; and they only employ as Journeymen, a Set of Men who they have picked up possessed of a sober Countenance, and a solemn melancholly [*sic*] Face, whom they pay at so much a Jobb.[23]

The idea that someone's business is 'to watch Death' is a grim one, but it was one that informed a lot of the more satirical and critical imagery of the eighteenth-century undertaker. Figures like 'Strip-Corps, the Dead-Monger' appear in satirical pamphlets in the eighteenth century, with illustrations of ghoulish undertakers preying on the nearly deceased like a pack of vultures.[24]

As can be seen by Greenhill's dismissal of undertakers as 'quacks', the profession most associated with 'appropriate' embalming was that of the surgeon. While an apothecary could carry out some procedures to slow down the signs of decay, it was the surgeon who could truly arrest decomposition.

Greenhill, who was himself a surgeon, dedicated *Νεκροκηδεια* [*Nekrokideia*, funeral], his book on the 'Art of Embalming', to Hans Sloane, a physician who served three monarchs, Anne, George I and George II. Sloane, like a number of surgeons and physicians, experimented with methods of embalming, but, on the whole, these were variations on the technique of evisceration, inserting herbs into incisions on the body and immersing the corpse in alcohol or some other preservative fluid. These were tried and tested techniques after all, as they had been used on members of the royal family for centuries. Sometimes, they achieved amazing results, with the body of Cnut II, who died in 1042, still looking pretty good when it was discovered in Winchester Cathedral in 1776. Other times, the results were not so good, as when the corpse of Henry I was brought into Reading Abbey in 1136, it was said that the 'strong, prevalent stench' was so bad that it killed a man.[25]

It goes without saying that the cost of embalming was dependent on which of the professions you employed to carry out the task. Although records are patchy for lower-class funerals, information about the funerals of monarchs who died during and shortly after Hannah Beswick's lifetime are illuminating. When Mary II died in 1694, her body was handled by an apothecary, at a cost of £200. But when George II died in 1760, and his body was preserved by surgeons, the cost was £433 13s.[26]

Although Hans Sloane and other medical men had experimented with techniques for preserving the human corpse in the late seventeenth and early eighteenth centuries, it was only in the 1770s that a new and innovative method was proposed. Anatomist and surgeon William Hunter proposed a method for embalming the body that utilized the circulatory system to introduce preservative chemicals into the body, rather than inserting substances into incisions.

But wait – we already know this.

The method of embalming proposed by William Hunter was not only a way for an anatomist to demonstrate the way the arteries and veins worked, it was also a process that would alter the practice of funereal preservation. It is still used for funerals today. For example, the very tasteful and gentle description of embalming offered on the website of Coop Funeralcare reads:

> Embalming is a process where natural fluids of the body are replaced (via the arterial system) with a solution to help preserve, sanitise and improve the appearance of the person who has died. The solution is a combination of formaldehyde, natural oils, colourants and water, which help restore the appearance of the skin.[27]

This is Hunter's technique, combined with the more modern requirements that mortuary services 'sanitise and improve the appearance' of a dead body, so that even an ordinary person can lie in state in their home, or in an open casket at their funeral.

* * *

So, what *did* Hannah want for her funeral? Did she want a triple-coffin burial with a hearse and some flamboys? Did she expect her family to hire an undertaker, a Strip-Corps with a sober countenance and a melancholy face? Did she want to be interred in an overflowing churchyard, stacked on top of the coffins of her parents and her brother, or in a vault that was already full to the brim with other members of her family?

Or was she more interested in the preservation of her physical body, to ensure it remained 'uncorrupted' and free from the dishonour of putrefaction and decay? Was she willing to pay a truly regal sum to a professional surgeon who could ensure this?

Embalming comes not out of a fear of being buried alive, but out of a fear of being buried dead. Accounts of medical and mortuary embalming, from Greenhill's in 1705 to the Coop's in 2023, are consistent in their claims that embalming will make a corpse more 'lifelike'. This might remind us of Faujas de Saint-Fond, gazing on the corpse of Miss Johnson and stating that she almost looked as though she were asleep. The idea of preserving the body as in life, keeping it free of the signs of death, is a powerful one.

The problem Hannah faced is that, in 1758, you could have a cutting-edge arterial embalming, or you could have a burial. You couldn't have both.

As we've seen from accounts of the techniques practiced by the Hunters and by John Sheldon, the new arterial preservation (or 'mummification' as it became known) required the prepared corpse to be dried out as well as embalmed. Once the viscera had been removed, and the preserving chemicals introduced into the veins and arteries, the body then had to be packed into a box with a desiccant substance, like plaster of Paris or chalk, and sealed up for several years while the process took effect.

At the same time, a death had to be registered (usually at the church) shortly after it occurred, with a burial arranged at the same time. No clergyman worth his salt is going to take the risk of registering a death and then taking the word of a surgeon that the experimental procedure he was trying out would be done in a few years, so could the burial wait until then, please? This is the reason, I suspect, why there were mummified bodies in the collections of the Hunters, John Sheldon and Charles White. They ceased to be 'manifestly useful objects' for teaching purposes almost immediately, but you couldn't just leave them at the local churchyard to be buried, and disposing of them any other way would be sacrilegious. All they could ever be was curiosities.

There are indications in Hannah's will that she was actively seeking to be embalmed by Charles White. The £400 for funeral expenses is one. The requirement that three women who were close to her remained at her home for the duration of several years is another. The discovery of the Ghastly Find in 1890 certainly suggests that some part of Hannah's body was kept separately and sealed up in a leaden box. And we know from accounts of other funerals that a viscera box need not be kept in the same place as the rest of the body.

Assuming the lead casket was a viscera box, we don't know what sort of ceremony was performed when it was put into the ground. Reports from 1890, working on the idea that it was some sort of grisly receptacle for a body-snatcher or a murderer, raise the question of why it was buried in a double-shelled coffin, using both wood and lead, neither of which were cheap materials. If this was a viscera box, and if

Hannah had instructed her close friends and family to conduct some sort of funerary rites for the part of her body that could not be preserved, then surely that's exactly what we would expect to see.

If Hannah Beswick truly was so afraid of being buried dead that she paid her friend, the eminent surgeon Charles White, to embalm her using a new technique he'd learnt in London, she may have been willing to sacrifice burial in a churchyard in her quest to remain an 'uncorrupted corpse'. Her heart (and other organs, but the heart is the most poetic) were buried, in sight of her friends and family, in a wooden coffin encased in lead. Her close companion Mary Greame would not only sit vigil over Hannah's body as it was slowly preserved in an airtight box, but would also live by the grave of Hannah's heart for the rest of her natural life.

Or until she married a lawyer and moved to Halifax, but let's not ruin the moment.

When he considered Hannah Beswick's afterlife as a museum exhibit, Francis Nicholson called it 'the ungenteel fate'. But was it really less genteel than having your rotting remains shoved into a shallow grave, at risk of being dug up again by a clumsy sexton? Or by the contractors hired to extend a tramline?

Let's compare Hannah Beswick to two other Manchester women called Hannah for a moment. In 1800, Hannah Rylance died at the age of ninety. She was buried in the graveyard of the Cross Street Chapel at a depth of just six inches, due to the number of other bodies beneath her. In 1827, Hannah Hatfield died at the age of seventy-three and was also placed in a grave that was full.

In 2014, both of these Hannahs were dug up when the graveyard was exposed during the construction of the 'Second City Crossing' for Manchester's Metrolink tram system. After lying in their graves as, presumably, they'd wanted, the two Hannahs – along with numerous other bodies at both Cross Street and the site of the old St Peter's Church, which was built between 1788 and 1794 close to where the Natural History Society would build its museum – suddenly became 'manifestly useful objects'. A tent went up around the site of the old cemetery, and the bodies were exhumed, studied, photographed and written about, because they 'provided an insight into life in Manchester before and during the Industrial Revolution'.[28] You can easily find pictures online of decomposed bodies (sanitized as fragments of bone, being carefully held by a studious osteologist), traces of rotted coffins, and fragments of decayed personal items that were buried with the bodies, as well as information about how many of the people exhumed smoked pipes, how many wore corsets and how many had rickets.

The names of Hannah Rylance and Hannah Hatfield are now associated with decomposition and decay, whereas the name of Hannah Beswick will only ever be associated with the continued preservation of her corpse.

Who really had an ungenteel fate? Hannah Beswick has been many things: a museum exhibit, a ghost, an urban legend, a neon sign in a trendy bar. But one thing she has never been is a rotted, corrupted corpse at the mercy of anyone with a spade.

13

Unremarkable

If this was a documentary, this would be the moment when the screen fades to black and writing appears informing you of what became of the people you've seen.

Hannah Beswick, of course, died in 1758 and was buried in Harpurhey Cemetery in 1868.

Charles White retired to Sale Priory, and in 1803 he suffered an attack of ophthalmia (inflammation of the eye), which left him blind. He died on 20 February 1813. He was buried at St Martin's Church in Ashton-on-Mersey.

Mary Greame remained at Cheetwood Hall until 1767, when she married Halifax attorney Richard Hopwood. Mary was fifty when she married, and her husband was about a decade older, so there were no children. When Mary died, she left almost the entirety of her sizeable estate to the children of her sister Ann and her brother John. In particular, Mary left bequests to her niece Ann Greame, John's daughter, including possession of a property called Lower Wat Ing during her lifetime and the furniture Mary 'brought from Cheetwood'. Ann Greame would go on to become the second wife of John Scholefield Firth and stepmother to his daughter Elizabeth. Firth was a friend of the Brontës, and he and Ann would become godparents to Branwell Brontë in 1817.

Mary Greame died on 8 November 1788, and she was buried in Halifax Parish Church with her husband.

Esther Robinson, Mary's co-executrix and daughter of Hannah's cousin Thomas, would also marry a lawyer from Halifax. In 1769, Esther married William Prescott of Calico Hall, and became stepmother to his children by his first wife. In the same year, William was engaged by his brother-in-law, Robert Parker, to help deal with the problem of the so-called Cragg Vale Coiners, and he attended the enquiry called by the Marquis of Rockingham after the murder of William Deighton. William Prescott wasn't very good with money, and he ended up in serious debt by 1776. Robert Parker stepped in and bought Calico Hall to prevent it from being sold out of the family. William and Esther went to live in a house at Stump Cross that Parker owned, and the couple died around fourteen years later, within two weeks of each other.

Esther Robinson died on 12 December 1791, and she was buried in the Holdsworth Chapel of Halifax Parish Church with her husband and other members of the Prescott family.

Thomas Robinson, Esther's younger brother, inherited Birchen Bower. He married Elizabeth Kay of Bury, and their son Joshua Kay Robinson inherited the property on his father's death. Joshua married Ann Whitehead, and they had a number of children at Birchen Bower.

Joshua Kay Robinson died in 1828, at the age of just forty-one. He was buried at St Margaret's Church in Hollinwood.

Joshua's eldest son, James Robinson, moved to the United States. He died on 29 March 1850, at the age of forty, and was buried at Christiana Church cemetery in Newark, New Castle County, Delaware. Joshua's eldest daughter was named Hannah Beswick Robinson, and she married Joseph Coates and moved to the Isle of Man. Hannah died at Beach Houses, Ramsey on the Isle of Man in February 1866.

In 1773, another beneficiary of Hannah's will, Esther Robinson's younger sister Ann, married a man named Thomas Pickering, who was a woollen-draper with a business at 8 Smithy-Door, near the Collegiate Church in Manchester. Thomas and Ann had five children: Elizabeth (Betty), Esther, John, Susannah and Samuel. John and Susannah died in infancy. Ann Pickering died in 1792, and her daughter Betty (aged twenty) died in 1796.

In 1793, Thomas Pickering declared bankruptcy and, a few years later, had to seek an alternative income for himself and his two surviving children, Esther and Samuel. While I can't be absolutely certain about what happened next, there's a tantalizing suggestion in an unexpected source.

In Samuel Bamford's *Passages in the Life of a Radical*, the author recounts some memories of childhood, specifically from the period when his father was working as the governor of a Manchester workhouse. Bamford recalls the death of the workhouse schoolmaster, Mr Rose, and writes:

> His place was filled by a Mr Pickering, who, like his predecessor, had been in business and failed. Mr Pickering was about fifty years of age, a quick and rather haughty kind of man, who endeavoured to maintain a remnant of the authoritative manner of his former state, though it was greatly out of place in the situation he then occupied. My father, I recollect, was under the necessity of setting him right once or twice, after which, as he came round to understand his position better, he was not an unpleasant associate. His wife had died some time before, leaving him two children, a son and a daughter, to provide for. The latter, who was a sweet-looking, affectionate young woman, probably from sixteen to eighteen years of age, lived in the family of a Mr Richardson, who kept a large glass and china shop at the top of Smithy Door: and the son, Samuel, who was a fine lad about my own age, and had a great resemblance of his sister, came to live with his father at the workhouse.[1]

Of course, it's possible that this isn't our Mr Pickering, but the similarities are incredibly striking.

Bamford goes on to describe how he and Sam Pickering would play together, especially imaginative games of 'sea-dangers, shipwrecks and lone islands' inspired by their favourite tale, *Robinson Crusoe*. Sadly, Sam Pickering would later decide to seek real-life adventure, and after his father's death, he 'went to sea' and 'was lost'.[2]

Bamford gives us no information about the fate of Sam's older sister. But I can furnish you with some. Esther Pickering remained in Manchester and never married. She died on 16 March 1844, at the age of sixty-seven. In her will, she left bequests to her servant, Harriet Street, and to Hannah Renshaw, the daughter of her cousin Esther Renshaw (née Robinson, sister to Joshua Kay Robinson). She also left £100 to the Manchester Infirmary, but I don't know if she knew she was following in her first cousin, twice removed's footsteps when she wrote this line in her will.

Esther Pickering died in 1844 and was buried in St John's Churchyard, near Byrom Street and Quay Street in Manchester.

All of these people lived their lives, which might perhaps be called unremarkable, and were dead before Hannah was buried. The legacies of Hannah's will, which took four lawyers to construct, had dwindled away, been sold or passed on to people that Hannah had never met, while her body was still a semi-anonymous museum exhibit. *Sic transit gloria mundi.*

* * *

There is another character that has played a key role in this story: the greatest village in England. It's only fair to see how Manchester progressed in the 110 years between Hannah's death and her burial.

Hannah died in a town, but was buried in a city. Manchester got its first MP in 1832, and its borough charter and town council in 1838. City status was granted in 1853.

We've already seen what became of Hollinwood and Cheetwood in the nineteenth century. King Street would also undergo a transformation, though it continued to be a fashionable and expensive area of town. By the beginning of the nineteenth century, the medical men had given way to bankers, with the Bank of England opening a branch on the street in 1845.

Charles White's house on the corner of King Street and Cross Street was demolished in the early 1800s. A new building was erected on the site in 1822–25, designed by architect Francis Goodwin in a Grecian style, and this would become Manchester's first town hall. Manchester, as ever, had ideas above its station, as the town hall was constructed before the borough charter was granted. From 1838, the building would house the Manchester Corporation and then, a little later on, Manchester Town Council. By 1863, the city had outgrown the building, and planning began for a new town hall – 'equal if not superior, to any similar building in the country' – on nearby Albert Square.[3] This new building was designed by Alfred Waterhouse, and the foundation stone was laid in October 1868. The old town hall on King Street was converted into a lending library, before becoming a branch of Lloyd's Bank. The building was eventually demolished in 1912 to make way for a new building in Edwardian Baroque style (now housing a pizzeria, dental clinic and boutique 'workplace solutions'), but the Grecian façade was preserved and relocated to Heaton Park, a municipal park in the north of the city (the former estate of the Earls of Wilton, and the location to which Satterfield's conveyed the body of the Countess of Wilton for her grand funeral in 1858).

Peter Street, which would house the museum in which Hannah was displayed from 1835, was constructed in 1794. St Peter's Church, on Mosley Street, was constructed around the same time. On 16 August 1819, Peter's Fields, the area just off Peter Street, was the site of a meeting of around 60,000 people who were campaigning for radical political reform. Samuel Bamford was there, as was James Brierley (father of Ben Brierley). The meeting ended in tragedy when local magistrates sent the Manchester and Salford Yeomanry to arrest Henry Hunt, who was addressing the meeting, and then the 15th Hussars to break up the crowd. Eighteen people died and hundreds were injured in the ensuing attack, which was dubbed the Peterloo Massacre by the *Manchester Observer*.

In the aftermath of Peterloo, the *Manchester Guardian* was founded (in 1821) as a direct response to the perceived bias in the press's reporting of events. In 1840, a wooden meeting hall was constructed on the site, and then a brick replacement was built in 1842. These halls would host further radical meetings, concerned with both parliamentary reform and, increasingly, the fight against the repressive Corn Laws. In 1853, the brick meeting hall was replaced with a new building (completed in 1856), known as the Free Trade Hall, funded by public subscription and operating as both a meeting place and a concert hall. The Free Trade Hall became the home of the Hallé Orchestra in 1858, and it would host a meeting in 1862 to discuss Manchester's response to the 'Cotton Famine' (the shortage of raw cotton caused by the blockade of the southern states in the American Civil War). As a result of the 1862 meeting, a group of Manchester men wrote a letter to Abraham Lincoln, which urged him to continue fighting for the abolition of slavery. The letter also claimed Manchester would continue to boycott slave-grown cotton, even in the face of economic difficulties.

In April 1868, a few months before Hannah Beswick was buried at Harpurhey, the Free Trade Hall was the venue for the first public meeting of the National Society for Women's Suffrage. The speaker at the meeting was Lydia Becker, a suffragist and scientist, whose family rented Foxdenton Hall in Chadderton, formerly the home of Robert Radclyffe, esq., one-time executor of Hannah's brother's will. About five or six years later, a teenager named Emmeline Goulden would attend another of Lydia Becker's meetings at the Free Trade Hall, which resulted in her committing herself wholeheartedly to the cause of women's suffrage. And a couple of years after that, Lydia Becker would introduce Emmeline to her friend Richard Pankhurst.

It may come as something of a surprise, but the first women to vote in general elections did so while Hannah Beswick's body was still on display at the Peter Street museum. Given that Hannah was born at a time when not only did Manchester have no political representation in parliament, but the country itself didn't even have a prime minister, it's almost unbelievable to imagine a woman (and a widowed shopkeeper at that) casting a vote in a general election before Hannah's body was in the ground.

In 1867, Lilly Maxwell of Chorlton-on-Medlock mistakenly appeared on the register of voters for a by-election. She was probably not the first woman to have found herself unexpectedly able to vote, but she was treated as a legal test case by Lydia Becker and her fellow campaigners. Lilly was escorted to the polling station, where she duly cast her vote. The following year, around a thousand women were able to exploit a legal loophole and vote in the general election. The loophole was closed shortly afterwards, despite legal challenges by Richard Pankhurst and other lawyers supportive of the cause, and it would be over fifty years before the next woman could vote in a general election.

The Free Trade Hall was separated from the Natural History Society's museum by another building – the Theatre Royal. This building was constructed in 1845 and run by John Knowles, who also made marble chimneypieces. The theatre on Peter Street replaced the previous Theatre Royal, on Fountain Street, which burnt down in 1844 (and which had, in its turn, replaced an earlier Theatre Royal on Spring Gardens, which had opened in 1775). In 1847, Charles Dickens performed at the theatre, in a production of *Every Man in His Humour*.

Both the Free Trade Hall and the Theatre Royal are still standing on Peter Street today. The former is now a Radisson Hotel, and the latter is a disused nightclub, remembered by some as the location of Take That's first ever TV appearance in the early 1990s. *Sic transit gloria mundi.*

* * *

The Manchester that Hannah was buried in was almost an entirely different place to the town that had existed in her lifetime. It's easy to fall into a sort of nostalgia when thinking about these changes, lamenting (as the newspapers did in 1890) the lost halls and villages of Manchester's past. However, there are any number of reasons why life for Mancunians in 1868 was preferable to that in 1758.

For one thing, smallpox was getting sorted. The development of a vaccination in the late 1790s, and its rollout in the early decades of the nineteenth century, was starting to have an effect. The death rate plummeted in Britain in the 1840s, and the vaccination became compulsory in 1853. There would be one final smallpox pandemic in the 1870s, with UK death rates shooting back up in 1871 and mandatory vaccination becoming enforced (parents who did not vaccinate their children in infancy faced fines or imprisonment), but this was the last major outbreak and UK smallpox deaths tailed off dramatically in the final decades of the century.

The work of scientists such as Louis Pasteur, who is often credited as the founder of bacteriology, introduced 'germ theory', leading to the prevention of bacterial infections and the development of vaccinations for rabies and anthrax, and antitoxins for diptheria.

In 1854, Florence Nightingale would arrive in what was then known as Constantinople to work as a nurse at a British army hospital. After her work to improve conditions at this hospital dramatically reduced the death rate, Nightingale would go on to help professionalize and transform nursing. She founded her first training school for nurses in 1860.

As well as medical developments, the years in which Hannah lay unburied saw all manner of inventions that would transform everyday life. Batteries, raincoats, balloons, staplers and traffic lights. Ice machines, sewing machines, safety pins, rotary washing machines and the principles of fibre optics. (Admittedly, machine guns, plastics and torpedoes as well, but it can't all be positive.)

As we've seen in earlier chapters, Manchester underwent some significant changes in terms of education in the nineteenth century as well, with the foundation of the Mechanics' Institute in 1824 and Owens College in 1851. While women could attend some public lectures – even as far back as the College of Arts and Sciences – most of these educational developments were intended for boys and men.

In 1862, Elizabeth Wolstenholme, a woman who, like Hannah Beswick, was born in Cheetham, joined the College of Preceptors (now the Chartered College of Teaching) with the intention of improving standards of primary school teaching for girls. Wolstenholme had been working as the headmistress of a private girls' boarding school for a number of years, despite having had limited formal education herself, and she was committed to improving the educational opportunities for girls in the city, and in the country. In 1865, Wolstenholme founded the Manchester branch of the Society for Promoting the Employment of Women, an organization set up in 1859 by Lydia Becker, Jessie Boucherett, Barbara Bodichon and Adelaide Anne Proctor to promote training and employment opportunities for women, and also the Manchester Schoolmistresses Association, an organization set up to support women teachers. Two years later, Wolstenholme would represent Manchester on the National Council for Promoting the Higher Education of Women.

The big successes of these organizations would come in the 1870s. The University of London awarded its first degrees to women in 1878, but there were some more local advances made before then. Manchester High School for Girls was founded in 1874, with the support of prominent members of Manchester society (including Robert Dukinfield Darbishire and his wife Harriet), and it was the first school in the north of England to offer a secondary curriculum for girls with an academic focus. And in 1877, the Manchester and Salford College for Women, an independent college with close links to Owens College, opened its doors to its first students, offering further education for 16–19 year olds with examinations supervised by Owens College staff.

Among the committee members of the new college was Meta Gaskell, daughter of novelist Elizabeth Gaskell, and Oliver Heywood, then president of the Manchester Mechanics' Institute.

Finally, if avoiding smallpox and getting a proper education aren't your thing, the public entertainment on offer in Manchester was far superior in 1868 than it had been in 1758 (when, you may recall, the town had only really had one public concert series and most people's social lives revolved around house calls and parties).

For example, Belle Vue Zoological Gardens, situated to the east of Manchester, opened in 1836. Originally constructed to house the aviary of part-time gardener John Jennison, who had previously opened his own gardens (called Strawberry Gardens) to the public before converting his house into a pub (called the Adam and Eve), Belle Vue was first intended as a set of formal gardens, with mazes, lakes and hothouses, for the enjoyment of the middle classes. In 1843, Jennison expanded one of the lakes, constructed an island in the middle of it, and opened a natural history museum on it. In 1858, he created an even larger lake, which had two paddle steamers that would take you around the lake for a penny, and by 1860 a menagerie was housed on the ground floor of the museum building.[4]

To the north of the town was Tinker's Gardens, also known as Vauxhall Gardens (copying the famous London pleasure gardens of the same name) or Elysium Gardens. Robert Tinker had run the Grape and Compass Coffee House in Collyhurst, near Harpurhey, in the late 1790s, but in the first decades of the 1800s, he changed both the name and the scope of his establishment. His new pleasure gardens offered space for promenading, music and dancing, as well as tea and other refreshments. In 1827, 50,000 people allegedly attended Tinker's Gardens to watch the ascent of a hot air balloon, but this may be apocryphal. What is more certain is that Tinker's Gardens was famous for its cucumbers, which grew particularly well due to the sandiness of the soil. One advertisement claimed that a cucumber had been grown that measured over seven feet in length and was, it was suggested, 'the greatest curiosity of the kind Nature ever produced in this kingdom'.[5]

* * *

Our story is in danger now of getting hijacked by vaccinations, degrees for women and giant cucumbers, all of which would have been entirely alien to Hannah Beswick.[6] Of course the city changed during the 110 years in which Hannah remained unburied – it could hardly be expected to stay the same.

However, this overview of the city's transformation isn't simply a whimsical tangent. I offer these examples because each of them has its roots (however difficult to discern) in the eighteenth century. The first lecture series open to women, the first attempts to inoculate against smallpox, the first public entertainments in the town, all occurred either during Hannah's lifetime or very shortly after her death.

My analysis of Hannah's will in an earlier chapter revealed a woman living on the border of the medieval and the modern, at a time of significant (if now often forgotten) change. This is a woman who, on the one hand, had to offer up a feudal tribute to a duke, but, on the other, chose to give a donation to the first major public health institution in the city. Hannah's life may have been pretty unremarkable, but the world she lived in wasn't.

Hannah's social and family networks brought her into contact with representatives of some of the oldest gentry families in the north of England – like the Radclyffes, who claimed a descent back to the Norman Conquest.[7] But they also connected her to families like the Robinsons, Kays and Gortons, whose family trees only become interesting in the 1700s. It's likely she spent most of her time at Cheetwood Hall, a Tudor manor house leased from an earl. But it's also likely she spent a lot of that time with the resolutely unmarried sister-in-law of a florist from Salford. And let's not forget Hannah's other house, a new-build property in the most fashionable part of town, surrounded by the homes of surgeons, scientists and non-conformists.

We have to come back to the one and only reason that the name of Hannah Beswick is still known today – her mummification. And that, too, can be viewed as a stepping stone between the old and the new worlds.

Hannah was a member of the landed gentry, a class identity that was becoming near enough obsolete while her body was still on display in Peter Street. Her class status, as well as some shrewd business decisions made by Hannah and various members of her family, resulted in a substantial disposable income. Like her grandfather before her, Hannah literally had bags of cash lying around her house, which she was free to spend on whatever she wanted. And yet, in her final wishes, she chose to use that money to pay a relatively young but already quite famous doctor to conduct an experimental embalming procedure that, while not really doing much to further the scientific study of anatomy in itself, would aid in the teaching and promotion of medical science in the decades to come.

I said in a previous chapter that we can't view Hannah in the same way as other preserved bodies that have been displayed in museums. Her story is not the same as that of Julia Pastrana or Saartje Baartman, for instance, and it has never (and will never) be treated to the same level of academic scrutiny as that of Asru. I'd suggest that this is because, when we look at it closely, the story of Hannah Beswick isn't the story of a museum exhibit at all. It's the story of a fairly ordinary woman who made an utterly extraordinary decision about her own body. It's no wonder that Hannah has always just been a curious footnote in academic studies of museums, because this was never really the story of how or why a museum decided to exhibit the Manchester Mummy. It was the story of Hannah Beswick, a Mancunian old maid, an eccentric testatrix and a true curiosity.

Epilogue

My local branch of Tesco – which would have been Hannah Beswick's local branch had she lived in a different time – opened in 2010, and it's built on the site of a graveyard.

In 2003, Manchester City Council granted planning permission for construction of a new supermarket on the site of the Cheetham Hill Wesleyan Cemetery on Thomas Street, just off Cheetham Hill Road (about a mile and a half from where Cheetwood Hall once stood). The Wesleyan Cemetery opened in October 1815, and it saw around 20,000 burials before its closure in 1968. The bodies in the cemetery were all exhumed in 2003 and buried in mass graves at St Peter's in Bury, the municipal Blackley Cemetery in North Manchester and Southern Cemetery in South Manchester. Descendants of the people buried in the Wesleyan Cemetery were told that reburial had to happen quickly, and so unless they were able to pay upfront for an individual grave, the bodies of their relatives would be reburied in mass plots in municipal cemeteries. In the end, the building of the supermarket took nearly seven years due to legal complications, meaning that families could have had time to raise funds for reburial after all. But it was too late. One angry family member described the experience on an internet forum in 2013: 'They gave no notice, just desecrated graves barely 80 years old.' He returned to post on the thread again in 2022: 'Tesco desecrated my Grandfather's Grave.'[1]

There's a small memorial garden in the corner of Tesco car park, which I've visited a few times while I've been writing this book. It's a reminder that, in the end, anyone can be unburied.

Epilogue

When I started researching the story of Hannah Beswick, I expected to spend a lot of time thinking about one woman who was kept out of the grave for over a century. And I have spent a lot of time thinking about her, of course. But I've also found myself thinking about a lot of other people who have been kept out, or taken from, their graves.

Like Hannah, the bodies of Saartje Baartman, Julia Pastrana, Maria van Butchell and Miss Johnson were not buried when the women died, but rather exhibited for decades in museums and shows. The skeleton of Charles Byrne, known as the Irish Giant, is still held in a museum collection, and it was only removed from public view in January 2023.

Asru and the unnamed (and now forgotten) Peruvian mummy who were housed in the Peter Street museum with Hannah were snatched from their graves after centuries, transported to another country and used for entertainment and education purposes. There is no plan to repatriate the body of Asru, nor does anyone seem to know the fate of the Peruvian body that was sold for nineteen shillings in 1868. There's more information available about the horse Vizir than about this anonymous person's mortal remains.

Lewis Brierley was taken from his grave in Mottram by anatomists in 1829. The head of John Brogan was taken by a medical student in 1832, his coffin weighted with a brick to conceal the desecration. The heads of Thomas Sydall and Thomas Deacon were removed from their bodies and displayed in St Ann's Square in 1745.

Bodies that went into graves as intended don't always stay there. Hannah Hatfield and Hannah Rylance – along with hundreds of other people buried at Cross Street Chapel – were exhumed to make way for Metrolink's 'Second City Crossing' tramline, just as hundreds of bodies were exhumed to make space for a Tesco car park in Cheetham Hill.

While the 'tinned salmon' remains found in Cheetham shocked and titillated newspaper readers in 1890, the story told in this book is full of body parts that have been preserved separately after the death of their owners. Whether it's the romantic story of Percy Shelley's heart, the pious gift of the Earl of Derwentshire's heart to a convent in Paris, or the garden interment of Sir William Temple's heart, the preservation of one organ in particular has a certain poetic power. But what of other organs, the corroded human liver on display in Charles White's medical cabinet or the one thousand cadaveric parts and disarticulated bones still held in the Hunterian Museum in London? Are these not also unburied human remains, kept out of the grave?

* * *

As well as thinking about bodies, I've thought about graves a lot while I've been writing this book. You might imagine that, after spending so much time trying to get to know her, I've visited Hannah's grave.

I haven't. I can't. Not really.

Hannah's grave was left unmarked in 1868. The story goes that this was a deliberate act to avoid grave-robbers or latter-day body-snatchers. More likely, it was to save the Commissioners money (they went for a cheap coffin, after all). Until recently, the location of the grave wasn't known.

Harpurhey Cemetery, now known as Manchester General Cemetery, is a municipal graveyard that was opened in 1837, shortly before Harpurhey was incorporated into Manchester. It was the largest burial space in the town for some time, offering consecrated ground for both Church of England and non-conformist burials. However, not all records for the cemetery have survived, so there are no official records for burials in consecrated ground prior to 1886. Many of the gravestones are now damaged or worn, making it hard to see what was once engraved upon them.

In 2010, a group of volunteers began the Manchester General Cemetery Transcription Project, dedicated to transcribing information from the surviving headstones and preserving the stories of some of the individuals buried in the cemetery. It is thanks to the work of these volunteers that we now know for certain that Harry Ludlam was correct in his 1966 assertion. Hannah was buried in plot C223 at the cemetery; however, we can only surmise where, exactly, that plot was.[2]

The Manchester General Cemetery Transcription Project reveals a lot about the impermanence of the grave. While a body might never be exhumed (either accidentally or deliberately), the site of its final resting place might be forgotten or obscured. So many of the gravestones in Manchester General Cemetery are illegible or beyond repair, as is the case in many graveyards around the country.

Epilogue

When there is no one left to visit or tend to a grave, when its location has all but been forgotten, does it still have any meaning?

* * *

I walk over the graves of unexhumed bodies every day on my way to work.

Hugh Hornby Birley, the magistrate and officer of the Manchester and Salford Yeomanry who led the cavalry into Peter's Fields on 16 August 1819 with an arrest warrant for Henry Hunt, died in July 1845 and was interred in his family's vault at St Peter's Church, just around the corner from the Natural History Society's museum.

The Birley family vault, along with numerous other vaults and graves, was unearthed during the construction of the St Peter's Square tram stop in 2015. Unlike with the Cross Street Chapel graveyard, the decision was taken to leave the human remains in their graves after examination, pave over them and put up a Metrolink stop. There is no indication that when you get off the tram here, you are walking over a grave site.

Manchester is full of sites like this. Hannah Beswick's parents, grandparents and younger brother were all buried at the Collegiate Church graveyard, which was the principal parish burial site at the time. This graveyard closed in 1848, after around 150,000 burials. A survey of existing gravestones was carried out in the nineteenth century, but as many were missing, illegible or badly damaged, this didn't tally with the number of people interred. The graves of Hannah's family were not recorded in this survey.

Most of the bodies in the Collegiate Church graveyard were never exhumed. They were just built over as the church became a cathedral and the area around it was developed. It feels like every time work is done at Manchester Cathedral, more old bodies are unburied. Most recently, in 2013, work to install a raisable dais in the nave unearthed five lead coffins and forty-nine bodies, which had been quietly residing in their final resting place for a couple of centuries.

If you've visited Manchester Cathedral for a service or a concert, you might well have walked over Hannah's mother's grave.

And if you've been to St John's Gardens near Quay Street, you might well have walked over the grave of Hannah's first cousin, twice removed, Esther Pickering. St John's graveyard closed in 1931 and the decision was taken to leave the bodies in place, flatten the headstones and cover them with eighteen inches of soil. St John's reopened as a public gardens in 1932. The only gravestone still visible is that of John Owens, the man whose legacy founded Owens College in 1851.

There are forgotten graves underneath our parks, shops and tram stops. But this should really come as no surprise, as this is a country where even a king can be found under a car park.

* * *

The story of Hannah Beswick encourages us to think about what it means to remain unburied, whether we approach this with a sense of the macabre, or through the academic lens of bioethics and museology.

But Hannah's story also encourages us to think about what it means to be buried. What is a funeral? What is a grave? Do we have a right to a 'final resting place'? And, if it's not to be final, who gets to decide if that resting place can be disturbed? The local authority? Tesco?

Is a grave still a grave when it's been forgotten?

Some of the more discomforting things I have talked about while telling Hannah's story – the accidental exhumations or desecrations by gravediggers, the unearthing of viscera during demolition works – reveal certain practicalities of burial practices that most of us would prefer not to think about. No one wants to think about the grave of a loved one being desecrated, and no one wants to imagine their own decomposing body making an unplanned reappearance.

The idea that an individual – or their family – has a right to determine how and when their body is disposed of on death is both emotive and deep-seated. We have just lived through a time when the spectre of mass graves (modern-day plague pits) was raised, albeit in more sensationalized media reports; among the many emergency powers included in the Coronavirus Act 2020 were some anticipating the possibility that 'local death management systems' could become overwhelmed. One of these gave local or national authorities the power to decide whether an individual was buried or cremated, even if that was at odds with the wishes of the individual or their family.[3] Among the many frightening things we experienced during COVID-19, the potential disruption of contemporary burial practices was certainly one of them, with unverified images of mechanical diggers preparing trenches for anonymous burials circulating on social media, like a twenty-first-century version of the cholera anxieties of 1831.

Again, this encourages us to think about why the grave is so important, and why we might feel so uncomfortable about the notion of an external body (a local or national authority, a landowner, a medical professional) determining how an individual's remains are treated on death. We might recall the Wool Act of 1667, which expressly forbade the use of linen shrouds (for economic reasons) in direct conflict with certain religious beliefs. Or the Murder Act of 1751, which gave ownership of a dead body to the anatomists, even when this went against the wishes of the deceased's family.

And yet …

The story of Hannah Beswick also reminds us that unburied bodies (whether left out of the grave or removed from it) are also a source of fun and entertainment.

I began this book by recounting my first experience of Hannah's story – a fun local ghost story to tell at Halloween. As I write this epilogue, Halloween is once again approaching, and the houses on my street are beginning to be decorated with images of skeletons, mummies, vampires and ghosts. One of my neighbours has fashioned a mock body out of a stuffed bin bag wrapped in strips of parcel tape, and hung on a string from an upstairs window. In my kitchen is a packet of 'Dried Mummy Brains', which is not – I hasten to add – corpse medicine, but a rather pleasant camomile tea made by Monster Mash Teas, a small business who specialize in horror-themed brews.

In the tales we tell at Halloween (or the rest of the year, if we're so inclined), the grave becomes a location of thrilling terror rather than existential trauma. Dracula, after all, is risen from the grave. And death is only the beginning. Burke and Hare are the subject of a 'macabre comedy' starring Simon Pegg and Andy Serkis, and let's not get started on the many representations of Igor, stealing body parts from fresh graves for Dr Frankenstein's experiments.

As I explored in the final chapter of Part I, Hannah's story is rarely told now with any sense of trauma related to the unburied body, just as her displayed corpse doesn't appear to have provoked any distress during its time as a museum exhibit. It's a curious tale, illustrated with gleefully ghoulish pictures of disinterred corpses, often told with tongue-in-cheek humour or a spooky whisper.

In the end, these two ways of thinking about death and the grave coexist in popular and academic culture. We hold anxieties about the post-mortem treatment of corpses alongside entertaining tales of post-mortem reappearance. Perhaps the latter is really just a way of dealing with the former.

Note for genealogists

If you have experience of researching a family tree, then you'll know that you spend just as much time ruling things out as ruling them in. For this reason, I've chosen not to list *all* of the sources I used to determine Hannah Beswick's family tree, because a lot of the records were consulted in order to test theories that turned out to be incorrect. Please do trust that I *did* consult these records, and I did consider alternative versions of Hannah's family until I settled on what I believe is the correct genealogy.

Below is a list of the key records I used to tell Hannah's story, once I'd identified which records actually did refer to her family. It is not exhaustive, but it should give you some clear starting points if you are also researching the Beswick and Robinson family trees.

Hannah Beswick's baptism was registered on 10 February 1694 at the Collegiate Church in Manchester (now Manchester Cathedral). Her will, dated 31 March 1758, and associated probate documents (including the inventory drawn up in July 1761) is held at Lancashire Archives. There is, of course, no record of Hannah's death.

Hannah's paternal grandfather (John Beswick) died in 1685, and his will, dated 18 June 1685, is held at Lancashire Archives. Hannah's paternal grandmother (Hannah Beswick) was buried on 9 June 1702 at the Collegiate Church. She died intestate, but a probate record for her estate, dated 8 August 1702, is held at Lancashire Archives.

Hannah's father (John Beswick) died in 1706. His will, dated 20 April 1706, is held at Lancashire Archives. Her half-brother (also John Beswick) was buried at the Collegiate Church on 14 October 1737. His will, proved on 8 May 1738, is held at Lancashire Archives.

Note for genealogists

Hannah Hadfield married John Beswick on 24 August 1693 in Mottram-in-Longdendale. She was buried at the Collegiate Church on 7 November 1695. Her father (Hannah's paternal grandfather), Thomas Hadfield, died in 1697. He was buried at St Michael and All Angels in Mottram-in-Longdendale on 4 April 1697. His will, dated 27 October 1697, is held at Cheshire Archives.

I was unable to find a record of Patience Buckley's marriage to John Beswick, but I have to assume it took place given subsequent records. Patience Beswick (née Buckley) married John Shaw at Saddleworth on 16 April 1713. She was buried in Bradford on 23 November 1717. Her husband John was buried on 14 December 1717, and his will, dated 1717/18, is held at the Borthwick Institute for Archives at the University of York. Patience's mother, Mary Buckley, left a will, dated 4 April 1725, and this is held at Lancashire Archives.

I looked through a large number of records to work out the Robinson family, including a number of public family trees posted on genealogy websites. Some key records for this particular story are: the marriage of Mary Robinson to John Whittaker at Blackley on 13 June 1747; the marriage of Esther Robinson to William Prescott at Halifax on 19 January 1769; and the marriage of Ann Robinson to Thomas Pickering at Manchester on 15 April 1773. Also significant are the wills of Joshua Kay Robinson (dated 29 December 1828) and Esther Pickering (dated 7 June 1844), which are held at Lancashire Archives, and of James W. Robinson (died 29 March 1850), which is held at Delaware County Register of Wills.

Charles White died in 1813. He was buried at Ashton on 1 March 1813. His will, dated 28 November 1811, is held at Cheshire Archives.

I've noted some of deductions I had to make about Mary Greame's family in the chapter where I discuss it. Mary married Richard Hopwood in Manchester on 18 May 1767, and her husband was buried on 26 May 1769. Mary's will was dated 19 September 1788 (and proved on 28 March 1789), and it's held at the Borthwick Institute for Archives at the University of York. Mary was buried at Halifax on 14 November 1788, thirty years after Hannah's death.

Notes

THE CABINET OF INSECTS

1 'Sale of the Valuable Library, &c.', *Manchester Mercury*, 18 October 1814, p. 1.
2 Samuel J. M. M. Alberti, 'Placing Nature: Natural History Collections and Their Owners in Nineteenth-Century Provincial England', *The British Journal for the History of Science*, 35:3 (September 2002), 291–311 (294).
3 Arnold Thackray, 'Natural Knowledge in Cultural Context: The Manchester Mode', *The American Historical Review*, 79:3 (June 1974), 672–709 (681).
4 Very little further information has survived about the career of Thomas Henry Robinson, though he does appear to have been involved in the foundation of the Manchester Academy (previously the Warrington Academy), a college for Unitarian students, in 1786. The college moved from Manchester to York in 1803, back to Manchester in 1840, and then to London in 1853. In 1880, it relocated to Oxford, and it survives as Harris Manchester College, Oxford, the smallest of the constituent undergraduate colleges of the University of Oxford.
5 Alberti, 'Placing Nature', 298.
6 Alberti, 'Placing Nature', 299.
7 'Manchester Natural History Society', *Manchester Courier*, 22 January 1825, p. 2.
8 'Manchester Natural History Society', *Manchester Mercury*, 8 November 1825, p. 3. There has been some confusion over the surname of the men who donated the Egyptian mummy to the Natural History Society. The current Manchester Museum, which continues to hold the mummy in its collection, gives the name 'Garrett' for the donors in some online resources. However, newspaper reports from 1825 clearly show that the surname was 'Garnett', and that they were gentlemen of the town. William Garnett (1782–1863) bought the Lark Hill estate in Salford, before moving to Quernmore Park in Lancaster (which remained in the possession of his descendants until 1990). Robert Garnett (1780–1852) bought Wyreside Hall in Dolphinhome, Lancashire.
9 'Manchester Natural History Society', *Manchester Courier*, 16 April 1825, p. 3.

10 Angela Stienne has written about some of the nineteenth-century 'unwrapping parties' that sat on the uneasy boundary between edification and entertainment. See Angela Stienne, *Mummified: The Stories Behind Egyptian Mummies in Museums* (Manchester: Manchester University Press, 2022), p. 109. Christina Riggs offers critical assessment of the significance of wrappings and unwrappings, through the lens of cultural and political history, in *Unwrapping Ancient Egypt* (London: Bloomsbury, 2014).

11 Karen Exell has written on modern perceptions of Asru and the ongoing discourse around the inclusion of human remains in the museum. See 'Covering the Mummies at the Manchester Museum: A Discussion of Individual Agendas Within the Human Remains Debate', in Howard Williams and Melanie Giles (eds), *Archaeologists and the Dead: Mortuary Archaeology and Contemporary Society* (Oxford: Oxford University Press, 2016), pp. 233–49; 'Domination and Desire: The Paradox of Egyptian Mummies in Museums', in Penelope Harvey (ed.), *Objects and Materials: A Routledge Companion* (London: Routledge, 2013), pp. 144–55. On the continuing controversies around Asru's unwrapped body in the popular press, see, for example, 'Sorry, Mummy, it's a Cover-up', *Manchester Evening News*, 18 April 2010, www.manchestereveningnews.co.uk/news/greater-manchester-news/sorry-mummy-its-a-cover-up-954406 [accessed 8 October 2023].

12 George Head, *A Home Tour Through the Manufacturing Districts of England, in the Summer of 1835* (London: John Murray, 1836), p. 76. Although Head's book mostly describes a tour he made in 1835, his trip to the King Street museum was made in the previous year.

13 Alberti, 'Placing Nature', 298.

14 Head, *A Home Tour*, p. 77.

15 Head, *A Home Tour*, p. 77.

16 Stienne, *Mummified*, p. 30.

17 See Richard Sugg, *Mummies, Cannibals and Vampires: The History of Corpse Medicine from the Renaissance to the Victorians* (London and New York: Routledge, 2011), p. 11. Recent studies have also explored the ways in which mummification was understood by Ancient Egyptians as a ritual, rather than an experiment or procedure: see Riggs, *Unwrapping Ancient Egypt*; Campbell Price, *Golden Mummies of Egypt: Interpreting Identities from the Graeco-Roman Period* (Manchester: Manchester University Press, 2023).

18 Head, *A Home Tour*, p. 78.

19 Stienne, *Mummified*, p. 138.

20 Head, *A Home Tour*, p. 78.

21 William Crawford Williamson, *Reminiscences of a Yorkshire Naturalist* (London: George Redway, 1896), p. 60.

22 Williamson, *Reminiscences*, p. 60.

23 For a description of these hoaxes, see Williamson, *Reminiscences*, pp. 66–7.

24 Francis Nicholson, 'The Old Manchester Natural History Society and its Museum', in *Memoirs and Proceedings of the Manchester Literary and Philosophical Society (Manchester Memoirs)*, vol. 58 (1913–14) (Manchester: Manchester Literary and Philosophical Society, 1915), pp. 1–15 (p. 3).

25 Nicholson, 'The Old Manchester Natural History Society', p. 3.

26 Oliver Goldsmith, *The History of The Earth and Animated Nature, With Copious Notes and an Appendix by Captain Thomas Brown*, edited by Thomas Brown (Glasgow: A. Fullarton and Co., 1832).

27 Annual Reports, 1840–1867. Manchester Museum Archive. University of Manchester Library. GB 133 MMA/1/5.

28 Annual Reports, 1840–1867. Manchester Museum Archive. University of Manchester Library. GB 133 MMA/1/5.

29 Benjamin Love, *Manchester As It Is* (Manchester: Love and Barton, 1839), pp. 124–5.

30 Thomas Ashton, *Visits to the Museum of the Manchester Natural History Society* (Manchester: Manchester Natural History Society, 1857), pp. 24–48.

31 Annual Reports, 1840–1867. Manchester Museum Archive. University of Manchester Library. GB 133 MMA/1/5.

32 See 'Free Family Activities All Summer', *Manchester Museum*, www.museum.manchester.ac.uk/event/summer-of-stories/ [accessed 8 October 2023].

33 Annual Reports, 1840–1867. Manchester Museum Archive. University of Manchester Library. GB 133 MMA/1/5.

34 Annual Reports, 1840–1867. Manchester Museum Archive. University of Manchester Library. GB 133 MMA/1/5.

35 Annual Reports, 1840–1867. Manchester Museum Archive. University of Manchester Library. GB 133 MMA/1/5.

36 Annual Reports, 1840–1867. Manchester Museum Archive. University of Manchester Library. GB 133 MMA/1/5.

37 Johann Georg Kohl, *England, Wales and Scotland* (London: Chapman and Hall, 1844), p. 130.

38 Nicholson, 'The Old Manchester Natural History Society', pp. 11–12.

BEHIND THE GIRAFFE

1 Annual Reports, 1840–1867. Manchester Museum Archive. University of Manchester Library. GB 133 MMA/1/5. This Mr Stubbs may be the 'J.S. Stubbs, esq.', a businessman, banker and landowner, who contributed various items and paintings for an exhibition at the Manchester Mechanics' Institute in 1842–43; see *Catalogue of the Fourth Exhibition at the Manchester Mechanics' Institution, Cooper Street, Christmas, 1842–3: With the Names of the Contributors* (Manchester: Cave and Sever, 1843).

2 Kohl, *England, Wales and Scotland*, p. 130.

3 Kohl, *England, Wales and Scotland*, pp. 130–1.

4 Joseph Crawford, '"A Tale of Plague": Anti-Medical Sentiment and Epidemic Disease in Early Victorian Popular Gothic Fiction', in Nicole C. Dittmer and Sophie Raine (eds), *Penny Dreadfuls and the Gothic: Investigations of Pernicious Tales of Terror* (Cardiff: University of Wales Press, 2023), pp. 114–36 (p. 115).

5 On the popularity of the medical profession in Manchester at this time, see Katherine Webb, '"The Most Stupid Place Under the Sun": Medical Practice and Professional Aspirations in the Industrial Town, 1820–60', *Bulletin of the John Rylands Library*, 87:1 (March 2005), 57–87.

6 Wendy Moore, *The Knife Man: Blood, Body Snatching, and the Birth of Modern Surgery* (New York: Broadway Books, 2005), p. 36.
7 Crawford, 'A Tale of Plague', p. 117.
8 Dean Kirby, *Angel Meadow: Victorian Britain's Most Savage Slum* (Barnsley: Pen and Sword Books, 2016), p. 36.
9 Kirby, *Angel Meadow*, p. 37.
10 Report from the Select Committee of the House of Commons on Anatomy, Evidence of Astley Cooper, cited in Moore, *The Knife Man*, p. 40.
11 William Chadwick, *Reminiscences of a Chief Constable* (Manchester: John Heywood, 1900).
12 Williamson, *Reminiscences*, p. 72.
13 Williamson, *Reminiscences*, pp. 72–3.
14 See Kirby, *Angel Meadow*, pp. 36–8.
15 See Thackray, 'Natural Knowledge', 684.
16 Nicholson, 'The Old Manchester Natural History Society', pp. 9–10.
17 Inventory, 1845. Manchester Museum Archive. University of Manchester Library. GB 133 MMA/1/6/3; Inventory, 1849. Manchester Museum Archive. University of Manchester Library. GB 133 MMA/1/6/4.
18 Ashton, *Visits to the Museum*, p. 2.
19 Ashton, *Visits to the Museum*, pp. 40–1.
20 Ashton, *Visits to the Museum*, p. 41.
21 Ashton, *Visits to the Museum*, p. 42; original emphasis.
22 Interestingly, Reynolds's long-running publication not only created one of the most grotesque and terrifying depictions of a body-snatcher, but also went on to humanize the figure, giving him the name Anthony Tidkins and a back-story that, while not excusing his crimes, certainly makes us ask whether society isn't a bit to blame.
23 Jan Bondeson, *Buried Alive: The Terrifying History of Our Most Primal Fear* (London and New York: W. W. Norton and Co., 2001).
24 Bondeson, *Buried Alive*, p. 208.
25 Bondeson, *Buried Alive*, pp. 124–6.
26 Jeremy Stern, 'A Tale Worthy of Poe: The Myth of George Bateson and his Belfry', *History News Network*, 28 October 2013, https://historynewsnetwork.org/article/153726 [accessed 8 October 2023].
27 Bondeson, *Buried Alive*, p. 87. Bondeson suggests that the bequest was '20,000 guineas' and includes further details that will become familiar when we turn our attention to later accounts of the case.
28 Edith Sitwell, *English Eccentrics* (London: Faber & Faber, 1958 [1933]), p. 17.
29 Thomas de Quincey, *Selected Writings of Thomas de Quincey*, edited by Philip van Doren Stern (New York: The Modern Library), pp. 289–90. The phrase 'all the races of men' refers to White's book *An Account of the Regular Gradation in Man*, to which I will return later in the story.
30 de Quincey, *Selected Writings*, pp. 292–4.
31 Peter Kitson, 'The Strange Case of Dr White and Mr De Quincey: Manchester, Medicine and Romantic Theories of Biological Racism', *Romanticism*, 17:3 (October 2011), 278–87 (278).

Notes

THE UNGENTEEL FATE

1 Barthélemy Faujas de Saint-Fond, *Travels in England, Scotland, and the Hebrides; Undertaken for the Purpose of Examining the State of the Arts, the Sciences, Natural History and Manners in Great Britain* (London: James Ridgeway, 1799), vol. 1, p. 40.
2 Faujas de Saint-Fond, *Travels*, pp. 42–3.
3 Faujas de Saint-Fond, *Travels*, pp. 43–4.
4 Faujas de Saint-Fond, *Travels*, p. 46.
5 Faujas de Saint-Fond, *Travels*, p. 47.
6 Advertisement, *St James's Chronicle*, 21 October 1773.
7 *Catalogue of the Contents of the Museum of the Royal College of Surgeons in London*, Part VI (London: R. Taylor, 1831), p. 55.
8 See Rachel Holmes, *The Hottentot Venus: The Life and Death of Sarah Baartman* (London: Bloomsbury, 2007).
9 *The Times*, 12 December 1811, p. 3.
10 *Catalogue of the Contents of the Museum*, pp. 54–55.
11 'Extraordinary Peruvian relic: just arrived and now exhibiting at the late Mr. Youngs office High St. Rochester: the entire body of a Peruvian woman, perfect as when in life; supposed to have been buried alive at the remote period of 500 years ago'. Between 1830–1840?. Wellcome Collection. Freak Shows Ephemera Box 5. Online. https://wellcomecollection.org/works/vt85m4xg [accessed 8 October 2023].
12 Stienne, *Mummified*, p. 138.
13 'Extraordinary Peruvian relic'.
14 'Leaflet advertising an exhibition of the mummified corpse of Julia Pastrana at the Burlington Gallery, 191 Piccadilly, London'. 1862? Wellcome Collection. Freak Shows Ephemera Box 3. Online. https://wellcomecollection.org/works/au8qz3hf [accessed 8 October 2023].
15 For a full account of the legal case, see Holmes, *The Hottentot Venus*, pp. 91–109. The 'Irish Giant' evoked here may well be Charles Byrne, who 'performed' in sideshows at the same time as Baartman. I will return to Charles Byrne later on in the story.
16 *The Baltimore Sun*, 10 November 1855, p. 1.
17 Harriet Beecher Stowe, 'The Woman Question', in *Hearth and Home* (1869), cited in Joan D. Hedrick, *Harriet Beecher Stowe: A Life* (New York: Oxford University Press, 1994), p. 360.
18 G. F. Cruchley, *Cruchley's London in 1865: A Handbook for Strangers, Showing Where to Go, How to Get There, and What to Look At* (London: G. F. Cruchley, 1865), cited in Lee Jackson, *The Dictionary of Victorian London*, www.victorianlondon.org/health/lockhospital.htm [accessed 8 October 2023].
19 Thomas Pettigrew, *A History of Egyptian Mummies, and an Account of the Worship and Embalming of the Sacred Animals by the Egyptians; with Remarks on the Funeral Ceremonies of Different Nations, and Observations on the Mummies of the Canary Islands, of the Ancient Peruvians, Burman Priests, etc.* (London: Longman, Rees, Orme, Brown, Green and Longman, 1834), pp. 258–9.

20 Pamphlet produced by the Royal College of Surgeons (apparently), cited in *Household Words*, 5 September 1857.
21 'Butchell, Martin van (1735–1812?)', *Dictionary of National Biography*, vol. 8 (1885–1900).
22 Charles Darwin, *The Variation of Animals and Plants Under Domestication*, vol. II (London: John Murray, 1868), p. 328.
23 Ashton, *Visits to the Museum*, p. 41.
24 Head, *A Home Tour*, p. 77.
25 Nicholson, 'The Old Manchester Natural History Society', p. 12.

WHAT WAS HER NAME?

1 Annual Reports, 1840–1867. Manchester Museum Archive. University of Manchester Library. GB 133 MMA/1/5.
2 Samuel J. M. M. Alberti, *Nature and Culture Objects, Disciplines and the Manchester Museum* (Manchester: Manchester University Press, 2012), p. 15. See also Leucha Veneer, 'How Manchester Museum Joined Arguing Societies Together', *BBC*, 27 October 2010, http://news.bbc.co.uk/local/manchester/hi/people_and_places/history/newsid_9132000/9132849.stm [accessed 8 October 2023].
3 Annual Reports, 1840–1867. Manchester Museum Archive. University of Manchester Library. GB 133 MMA/1/5.
4 Nicholson, 'The Old Manchester Natural History Society', p. 10.
5 Annual Reports, 1840–1867. Manchester Museum Archive. University of Manchester Library. GB 133 MMA/1/5; original emphasis.
6 Nikolaus Pevsner, *Lancashire I: The Industrial and Commercial South* (London: Penguin Books, 1969), p. 265.
7 See, for example, 'Manchester – Proposed Museum', *Bell's New Weekly Messenger*, 31 August 1845, p. 2.
8 Annual Reports, 1840–1867. Manchester Museum Archive. University of Manchester Library. GB 133 MMA/1/5.
9 Alberti, *Nature and Culture*, p. 20.
10 Annual Reports, 1840–1867. Manchester Museum Archive. University of Manchester Library. GB 133 MMA/1/5; original emphasis.
11 Later in the nineteenth century, Manchester Corporation would indeed construct a museum in Queen's Park, constructing a Gothic-style building in 1883–84 for the purpose of housing art for the public benefit. The Queen's Park Gallery was open to the public until the second half of the twentieth century. The building is currently not open to the public, but it survives as a conservation studio and storage site for the Manchester Art Gallery.
12 Annual Reports, 1840–1867. Manchester Museum Archive. University of Manchester Library. GB 133 MMA/1/5.
13 Bexwyke is a variant spelling of Beswick. The contribution of Hugh and Joan Bexwyke to the foundation of Manchester Grammar School is acknowledged in the present day by the 'Bexwyke Society', a name given to the group of people who have endowed a bursary place in perpetuity by donating the sum of £400,000 or more to the school. Joan Bexwyke (née Oldham) was Hugh Oldham's sister, and the wife of Robert Bexwyke, whose father Richard

endowed the Jesus chantry chapel at the Manchester Collegiate Church. As a widow in 1515, Joan had the economic agency to stand as a founder of Manchester Grammar School in her own right, alongside (but not subsumed into) her brother and son.

14 'The History of MGS', *The Manchester Grammar School*, www.mgs.org/2015/the-history-of-mgs [accessed 8 October 2023].

15 'The History of MGS'.

16 Don't be fooled by the current logo of the University of Manchester, which was introduced in 2004 and includes the claim 'Est. 1824' to assert itself as an older institution than University College London. The 1824 establishment date refers to the oldest constituent part of what is now the University of Manchester – the Manchester Mechanics' Institute. The Mechanics' Institute was converted to the Manchester Technical School in 1883, later becoming the Manchester Municipal College of Technology and being renamed University of Manchester Institute of Science and Technology (UMIST) in 1966, and eventually becoming a completely autonomous university with degree-awarding powers in 1994. The College of Technology had operated on a partnership agreement with the Victoria University of Manchester since 1905, but it retained its independent status until the two institutions formally merged in 2004. Additionally, although the University of Durham received its royal charter in 1832, it is not counted as a 'modern' university, as it was a College of Divinity throughout the nineteenth century, and therefore more comparable to Oxford and Cambridge than the University of London.

17 Love, *Manchester As It Is*, p. 128.

18 'College of Arts & Sciences, Established at Manchester', *Manchester Mercury*, 29 July 1783, p. 4; original emphasis.

19 'College of Arts and Sciences', *Manchester Mercury*, 30 September 1783, p. 1.

20 'College of Arts and Sciences', *Manchester Mercury*, 10 October 1786, p. 4; original emphasis.

21 A. E. Musson and E. Robinson, 'Science and Industry in the Late Eighteenth Century', *The Economic History Review*, new series, 13:2 (1960), 222–244 (225).

22 William Henry, 'A Tribute to the Memory of the Late President of the Literary and Philosophical Society of Manchester', *Memoirs of the Literary and Philosophical Society of Manchester*, second series, vol. III (1819), 204–40 (225).

23 Henry, 'A Tribute', 224.

24 Thomas Campbell, *Reprint of Mr Campbell's Letter to Mr Brougham, on the Subject of a London University, which Appeared in The Times of Feb. 9: Together with Suggestions which Appeared in the April Number of the New Monthly Magazine* (London: Longman, Hurst, Rees, Orme, Brown, and Green, 1825), pp. 1–3.

25 Henry Buckley Charlton, *Portrait of a University, 1851–1951: To Commemorate the Centenary of Manchester University* (Manchester: Manchester University Press, 1951), p. 22.

26 Sir Alfred Hopkinson, cited in Charlton, *Portrait of a University*, p. 27.

27 Charlton, *Portrait of a University*, p. 27.

28 See Chapter 1, n. 4 for information about the Manchester Academy.
29 Colin Lees and Alex Roberton, 'Early Students and the "University of the Busy": the Quay Street Years of Owens College, 1851–1870', *Bulletin of the John Rylands Library* (1997), 161–94 (163).
30 Lees and Roberton, 'Early Students', 163.
31 H. E. Roscoe, *Record of Work Done in the Chemical Department of the Owens College 1857–1887* (London: Macmillan, 1887), p. 9, cited in Lees and Robertson, 'Early Students', 169.
32 Lees and Robertson, 'Early Students', 171.
33 Lees and Robertson, 'Early Students', 185.
34 Bundle, 1868–1872. Manchester Museum Archive. University of Manchester Library. GB 133 MMA/1/8/3.
35 Nicholson, 'The Old Manchester Natural History Society', p. 14.
36 Minute Book, Jan 1868–10 Dec 1872. Manchester Museum Archive. University of Manchester Library. GB 133 MMA/1/8/1.
37 Note on Vizir, n.d. Manchester Museum Archive. University of Manchester Library. GB 133 MMA/1/9/4.
38 The body of Vizir is currently in a far better state than it was during its display in the nineteenth and twentieth centuries, as restoration and conservation work was carried out in 2016 following a successful campaign titled 'Sauvons Vizir [Let's Save Vizir]'. See 'Sauvons Vizir', *Le Blog des Actualités du Musée de l'Armée*, https://actualites.musee-armee.fr/feuilletons/sauvons-vizir/ [accessed 8 October 2023].
39 *Manchester Guardian*, 9 October 1868. The Burmese idol remained at Salford's Peel Park Museum until 1969, when it was returned to the Manchester Museum, in whose collection it remains today.
40 Minute Book, Jan 1868–10 Dec 1872. Manchester Museum Archive. University of Manchester Library. GB 133 MMA/1/8/1.
41 Letter Book, Feb 1868–Jul 1872. Manchester Museum Archive. University of Manchester Library. GB 133 MMA/1/8/2.
42 Letter Book, Feb 1868–Jul 1872. Manchester Museum Archive. University of Manchester Library. GB 133 MMA/1/8/2.
43 Letter Book, Feb 1868–Jul 1872. Manchester Museum Archive. University of Manchester Library. GB 133 MMA/1/8/2.
44 Letter Book, Feb 1868–Jul 1872. Manchester Museum Archive. University of Manchester Library. GB 133 MMA/1/8/2.
45 Letter Book, Feb 1868–Jul 1872. Manchester Museum Archive. University of Manchester Library. GB 133 MMA/1/8/2.
46 Letter Book, Feb 1868–Jul 1872. Manchester Museum Archive. University of Manchester Library. GB 133 MMA/1/8/2.
47 Letter Book, Feb 1868–Jul 1872. Manchester Museum Archive. University of Manchester Library. GB 133 MMA/1/8/2.
48 Letter Book, Feb 1868–Jul 1872. Manchester Museum Archive. University of Manchester Library. GB 133 MMA/1/8/2.
49 'A Curious Interment', *Manchester Guardian*, 15 August 1868.

Notes

MADAME BESWICK'S SUPERNATURAL PRANKS

1 James Dronsfield, *Ouselwood, or A Gathering of Old Chums* (Oldham: John Albinson, Ltd., 1921), pp. 112–13.
2 Dronsfield, *Ouselwood*, pp. 113, 116.
3 *Manchester Guardian*, 1 January 1877.
4 This threat continued into the twentieth century, with Manchester launching quite an aggressive campaign to incorporate Failsworth in the 1900s. A newspaper article at the time referred to Failsworth as 'the heiress whom Manchester and Oldham are wooing' (*Manchester Evening News*, 14 February 1914). Despite now being part of Greater Manchester, Saddleworth still proudly resists, with 'Welcome to Yorkshire' signs being displayed on the approach.
5 For a description of Hollinwood as a common, see Edwin Butterworth, *Historical Sketches of Oldham* (Oldham: J. Hirst, 1856), p. 6.
6 See Matthew Osborn, '"The Weirdest of All Undertakings": The Land and the Early Industrial Revolution in Oldham, England', *Environmental History*, 8:2 (April 2003), 246–69 (249).
7 Osborn, 'The Weirdest of All Undertakings', 249.
8 John H. Ingram, *The Haunted Homes and Family Traditions of Great Britain* (London: Gibbings & Co., 1897), p. 345.
9 Ingram, *Haunted Homes*, p. 351.
10 Ingram, *Haunted Homes*, p. 351.
11 Ingram, *Haunted Homes*, pp. 351–2.
12 Henry Frith, *Haunted Ancestral Homes*, edited by J. Murphy (Morrisville: Lulu.com, 2017).
13 'Authenticated Ghost Stories by Henry Frith', *Ripon Observer*, 16 January 1902, p. 3.
14 'Authenticated Ghost Stories by Henry Frith', p. 3.
15 'Authenticated Ghost Stories by Henry Frith', p. 3.
16 'Authenticated Ghost Stories by Henry Frith', p. 3.
17 'Authenticated Ghost Stories by Henry Frith', p. 3.
18 'Authenticated Ghost Stories by Henry Frith', p. 3.
19 *Middleton Guardian*, 29 June 1889.
20 *Middleton Guardian*, 13 July 1889.
21 *Manchester Guardian*, 1 January 1877.
22 There is a record of a John Beswick of Birchen Bower dying in 1737, and he left a will. There was also a John Beswick of Failsworth who joined the Pretender's army and played a part in the Jacobite rebellion in Manchester in 1745, who was executed for treason in 1746. Both of these Johns appear as Hannah Beswick's brother in different accounts of her family.
23 See, for example, *Runcorn Examiner*, 21 December 1889.
24 *Manchester City News*, 29 October 1904.
25 *Daily Herald*, 3 September 1931.

TINNED SALMON

1 'A Ghastly Find at Cheetham', *Middleton Guardian*, 5 July 1890, p. 8.

2 'A Ghastly Find at Cheetham', p. 8.
3 'A Ghastly Find at Cheetham', p. 8.
4 'A Ghastly Find at Cheetham', p. 8.
5 *Manchester Courier*, 4 July 1890.
6 *Manchester Times*, 22 August 1890.
7 *Manchester Times*, 5 July 1890.
8 Jan Harold Brunvand, *The Vanishing Hitchhiker: American Urban Legends and Their Meanings* (New York: W. W. Norton and Co., 1981) pp. xii, 4, xii, original emphasis.
9 *Manchester Times*, 22 August 1890.
10 *Manchester Guardian*, 1 January 1877.
11 Herbert W. Smith, 'The Manchester Mummy', in *Manchester Faces and Places*, xiv (March 1908), 126.
12 Smith, 'The Manchester Mummy', 126.
13 Smith, 'The Manchester Mummy', 126.
14 Smith, 'The Manchester Mummy', 126.
15 The walking guide for 'Sale Water Park and Priory Gardens' no longer appears on the Heritage Trees website, but it can be found as an uploaded file here: www.cityoftrees.org.uk/sites/default/files/AT_SaleWaterParkAndPrioryGardens.pdf [accessed 11 May 2023].
16 Folder: Charles White and Sale Priory, 1912–1949, n.d. Manchester Medical Collection: Biographical Files R-Z. University of Manchester Library. GB 133 MMC/2/WHITEC/2.
17 Folder: Charles White and Sale Priory, 1912–1949, n.d. Manchester Medical Collection: Biographical Files R-Z. University of Manchester Library. GB 133 MMC/2/WHITEC/2. As a side note, I can't help but note that Bosdin Leech paid £3 in 1934 for a partial transcript of Hannah Beswick's will. In 2022, I paid £11 for a series of high-resolution photographs of the full document, including probate details. I think I got the better deal.
18 Handwritten note on Smith, 'The Manchester Mummy'. Folder: Charles White and Sale Priory, 1912–1949, n.d. Manchester Medical Collection: Biographical Files R-Z. University of Manchester Library. GB 133 MMC/2/WHITEC/2.
19 Handwritten note on a cutting and typed transcript from *Manchester Guardian*, April 1935. Folder: Charles White and Sale Priory, 1912–1949, n.d. Manchester Medical Collection: Biographical Files R-Z. University of Manchester Library. GB 133 MMC/2/WHITEC/2.
20 Cllr A. H. Megson is probably best remembered (or only remembered) today as one of the founders of the Manchester and Cheshire Dogs' Home.
21 Folder: Charles White and Sale Priory, 1912–1949, n.d. Manchester Medical Collection: Biographical Files R-Z. University of Manchester Library. GB 133 MMC/2/WHITEC/2.
22 Folder: Charles White and Sale Priory, 1912–1949, n.d. Manchester Medical Collection: Biographical Files R-Z. University of Manchester Library. GB 133 MMC/2/WHITEC/2.
23 Folder: Charles White and Sale Priory, 1912–1949, n.d. Manchester Medical Collection: Biographical Files R-Z. University of Manchester Library. GB 133 MMC/2/WHITEC/2.

24 Folder: Charles White and Sale Priory, 1912–1949, n.d. Manchester Medical Collection: Biographical Files R-Z. University of Manchester Library. GB 133 MMC/2/WHITEC/2.
25 Folder: Charles White and Sale Priory, 1912–1949, n.d. Manchester Medical Collection: Biographical Files R-Z. University of Manchester Library. GB 133 MMC/2/WHITEC/2.
26 Folder: Charles White and Sale Priory, 1912–1949, n.d. Manchester Medical Collection: Biographical Files R-Z. University of Manchester Library. GB 133 MMC/2/WHITEC/2.
27 Folder: Charles White and Sale Priory, 1912–1949, n.d. Manchester Medical Collection: Biographical Files R-Z. University of Manchester Library. GB 133 MMC/2/WHITEC/2.
28 If Patience Buckley's name seems vaguely familiar to horror fans, that may be because (coincidentally) it is very similar to that of the murderous but tragic zombie redneck cannibal, Patience Buckner, in the film *The Cabin in the Woods*.
29 Sara Wasson, 'Gothic Cities and Suburbs, 1880–Present', in Glennis Byron and Dale Townshend (eds), *The Gothic World* (London and New York: Routledge, 2014), pp. 132–42 (p. 132).
30 'A Curious Corner of Manchester', *Manchester Times*, 14 June 1890, p. 5.
31 Smedley survived a little longer than Cheetwood, probably due to its distance from Manchester. It continued to be a place dominated by large houses and wealthy residents until the twentieth century, and a number of these large houses survive today (though some have been repurposed or split into smaller residences).
32 As you might have noticed, the Bury Old Road – in its modern incarnation – was indeed constructed *after* the Bury New Road. The reason for this curiosity of road naming is that Bury Old Road was a medieval route between Manchester and Bury that served the needs of ordinary people but proved difficult for commerce and trade vehicles. When a group of businessmen and merchants got together to discuss creating a turnpike trust, they decided to construct a 'new' road in 1826. By the end of the nineteenth century, the 'old' road had been (re)constructed.
33 'A Curious Corner of Manchester', p. 5.

MS BESWICK

1 Sitwell, *English Eccentrics*, p. 12.
2 'She's a Tall Farmyard Phantom', *Good Morning*, 3 February 1944, p. 1.
3 It's possible that the green skin tone was inspired by the marketing for another of Universal's monster movies – the 1931 *Frankenstein* starring Boris Karloff. There is a *Frankenstein* connection to the Hannah Beswick story, but it's very tangential and probably unexpected. John Leigh Philips, of cabinet of insects fame, was the son of John Philips who founded the company Philips and Lee with a man called George Augustus Lee. Lee lived in Smedley, now Cheetham Hill, with his sister, Harriet Lee who moved there after turning down a marriage proposal from William Godwin, Mary Shelley's father.

4 Harry Ludlam, *The Mummy of Birchen Bower and Other True Ghost Stories* (Slough: W. Foulsham and Co., 1985 [1966]), p. 17.
5 Ludlam, *The Mummy of Birchen Bower*, p. 18.
6 Ludlam, *The Mummy of Birchen Bower*, p. 18.
7 Ludlam, *The Mummy of Birchen Bower*, p. 21.
8 Ludlam, *The Mummy of Birchen Bower*, p. 24.
9 See, for example, Stienne, *Mummified*; Simon Chaplin, 'Dissection and Display in Eighteenth-Century London', in Piers Mitchell (ed.), *Anatomical Dissection in Enlightenment England and Beyond Autopsy, Pathology and Display* (London: Routledge, 2012), pp. 95–114.
10 See Jessie Dobson, 'Some Eighteenth Century Experiments in Embalming', *Journal of the History of Medicine and Allied Sciences*, 8:4 (October 1953), 431–41.
11 See, for example, David Castleton, 'The Manchester Mummy – How a Respectable English Woman Got Embalmed Egyptian Style', *The Serpent's Pen*, 9 December 2018, www.davidcastleton.net/manchester-mummy-hannah-beswick/ [accessed 8 October 2023].
12 Marco Margaritoff, 'How Hannah Beswick's Fear of Live Burial Turned Her into the Manchester Mummy', *All That's Interesting*, 4 January 2020, https://allthatsinteresting.com/manchester-mummy [accessed 8 October 2023].
13 'Myths of Manchester: The Curious Tale of the Manchester Mummy', *Manchester's Finest*, 12 September 2022, www.manchestersfinest.com/articles/manchester-myths-curious-tale-manchester-mummy/ [accessed 8 October 2023].
14 'Manchester Mummy', *Mummipedia*, https://mummipedia.fandom.com/wiki/Manchester_Mummy [accessed 8 October 2023].
15 'Manchester Mummy', *Wikipedia*, https://en.wikipedia.org/wiki/Manchester_Mummy [accessed 8 October 2023]. The 'Talk' page on the Wikipedia article for the 'Manchester Mummy' includes an interesting and rather rigorous debate from 2009 about the accuracy of some of the known 'facts' of the case. A discussion of the manner in which Miss Beswick's body was routinely inspected for signs of life by Dr White prompted one user, Malleus Fatuorum, to type a message simply reading, 'Bollocks'. This is reminiscent of the sentiment – if not the style – of E. Bosdin Leech's handwritten notes on the case from the 1930s.
16 'The Strange Fame of Hannah Beswick', *BBC*, 11 August 2009, http://news.bbc.co.uk/local/manchester/hi/people_and_places/history/newsid_8195000/8195234.stm [accessed 8 October 2023].
17 Shortly after the sign's appearance, it was revealed that it was made by businessman Frank Rothwell of Manchester Cabins. The following day, it was removed by the Highways Agency as it was considered a distraction for motorists. Anecdotally, I would add that a local myth circulated for a time that it was removed due to legal intervention from Hollywood.
18 See, for example, 'The Curious Tale of the Manchester Mummy'.
19 This story appears in E. M. Brockbank, *Sketches of the Lives and Work of the Honorary Medical Staff of the Manchester Infirmary, from its Foundation in 1752 to 1830 when it became the Royal Infirmary* (Manchester: Manchester

University Press, 1904), p. 11. Of course, it's quite likely apocryphal, but it gives an indication of how many powerful men in Manchester were known as 'confirmed Jacobites'.

20 'Exploring the Historic Street Names of Manchester', *Manchester's Finest*, 26 March 2020, www.manchestersfinest.com/manchester/exploring-the-historic-street-names-of-manchester/ [accessed 8 October 2023].

21 Cliff Goodwin, 'Sale of Manchester's Historic St George's House Confirmed', *Movehut*, 12 September 2014, https://news.movehut.co.uk/sale-of-manchesters-historic-st-georges-house-confirmed-23947/ [accessed 8 October 2023].

22 Miriam Bibby, 'Hannah Beswick, the Mummy in the Clock', *Historic UK*, n.d., www.historic-uk.com/HistoryUK/HistoryofBritain/Hannah-Beswick-The-Mummy-In-The-Clock/ [accessed 8 October 2023].

23 'Hannah Beswick', *Exhibition*, 20 October 2022, www.exhibitionmcr.co.uk/exhibition/hannah-beswick/ [accessed 8 October 2023].

24 Alan Thompson, 'Are You My Mummy?', *The Ratbag Encyclopedia*, 26 March 2017, www.warpedtime.com.au/encyclopedia/are-you-my-mummy/ [accessed 8 October 2023].

25 Sabrina, 'Unboxed and Unwrapped – Ripley's Mummy Collection', *Ripleys*, 29 April 2016, www.ripleys.com/weird-news/mummy-unboxing/ [accessed 8 October 2023].

26 'The Peculiar Afterlife of Ms Hannah Beswick', *TikTok*, 28 November 2022, www.tiktok.com/@livesandtimeshistory/video/7171078215832833286 [accessed 8 October 2023].

27 Dobson, 'Some Eighteenth Century Experiments in Embalming', 432.

HANNAH

1 Hannah is not the only descendant of Thomas Hadfield to gain notoriety. His great-great-grandson (Hannah's first cousin, twice removed) was John Hatfield (a variant spelling of Hadfield), who was executed in Carlisle in 1803 for forgery. John Hatfield was not only a forger, but a con artist who impersonated an MP. He is most notorious for his seduction of Mary Robinson, the 'Maid of Buttermere', a story that was written about by Wordsworth, Coleridge and, more recently, Melvyn Bragg. Thomas Hadfield is buried at St Michael and All Angels in Mottram, where, later, a gravestone would be erected to mark the empty grave of Lewis Brierley, whose body was stolen by anatomists.

2 The phrase 'dear and well-beloved children' appears in John Beswick's will.

3 Although some resources still claim that the Crumpsall Hall in which Humphrey Chetham was born was on the site now occupied by Crumpsall Park, this is incorrect. Crumpsall Old Hall, a post-medieval manor house, was closer to Cheetham Hill, near what is now Humphrey Street. In 1825, the new owners of the Crumpsall Hall estate, John and Thomas Blackwall, knocked down the old hall and built a new one further into Crumpsall. The new hall stood on the site that is now Crumpsall Park.

4 By the eighteenth century, Kersal Moor races offered a particular delight: nude male races, where women allegedly used the occasion to study the 'form' of potential marriage partners. The owner of Kersal Cell in the early eighteenth

century, poet John Byrom, was opposed to racing, but only succeeded in getting the Kersal Moor races stopped in 1746. They started again in 1750.

5 Elizabeth Byrom, *The Journal of Elizabeth Byrom in 1745*, edited by Richard Parkinson (Manchester: Chetham Society, 1857), p. 3.

6 Richard Kay (1716–1751), Diary, 1737–1751. Chetham's Library. Manchester. A.7.76. Excerpts of the diary are published in Richard Kay, *The Diary of Richard Kay, 1716–51 of Baldingstone, Near Bury: A Lancashire Doctor*, edited by W. Brockbank and F. Kenworth (Manchester: Chetham Society, 1968).

7 Virginia Brookes (ed.), *Priscilla Bunbury's Virginal Book* (Albany: PRB Productions, 1993); Howard Ferguson (ed.), *Anne Cromwell's Virginal Book, 1638* (Oxford: Oxford University Press, 1974); George Sargent (ed.), *Elizabeth Rogers' Virginal Book, 1656* (Muenster: American Institute of Musicology, 1971).

8 Occasionally, you might find the claim that Patience was pregnant at the time of John's death and subsequently bore another child (often called Wright). This isn't the case – John made a provision in his will *in case* Patience was pregnant at the time of his death, but there's absolutely no evidence that she actually was.

9 The office of 'prime minister' wasn't constitutionally recognized until much later, but it is generally agreed that Walpole was the first *de facto* prime minister.

10 Daniel Defoe, *A Tour Thro' the Whole Island of Great Britain, Divided into Circuits or Journies* (London: JM Dent and Co, 1927), Letter X. To the chagrin of Mancs across the ages, this letter from Daniel Defoe also described Liverpool as 'one of the wonders of Britain'.

11 The bequest made by Humphrey Chetham to found Chetham's Library would be worth, roughly, £1.5 million in today's money. And this was only one of the bequests in his will.

12 See Peter Maw, 'Provincial Merchants in Eighteenth-Century England: The "Great Oaks" of Manchester', *The English Historical Review*, 136:580 (June 2021), 568–618.

13 Cross Street Chapel is still in existence at this location; however, its present building was constructed in 1958, as the original building was destroyed in a bombing raid in 1940.

14 James's Square led into the street that became known as King Street in the 1740s. It is commonly held that the name 'King Street' was given to the thoroughfare in 1745, after the defeat of the Jacobite rebels.

15 Peter Arrowsmith. The Medieval Cultural Quarter, Manchester: An Archaeological Desk-Based Assessment. A Report for Chetham's School of Music, Manchester Cathedral and Manchester City Council. 2011. https://chethamsschoolofmusic.com/app/uploads/sites/2/2016/09/Part-1–Text.pdf [accessed 8 October 2023], pp. 35–6.

16 H. Harvey, 'Hannah Beswick and Her Bequests', *Oldham Chronicle*, 11 January 1958.

Notes

SUNDRY ODD THINGS

1 *Manchester Times*, 6 December 1834.
2 *Manchester Courier*, 12 October 1839.
3 Hannah Beswick Coates (née Robinson) died in 1866 in Ramsey on the Isle of Man. She was buried two years before her namesake, who had died 108 years earlier.
4 Samuel's cousin Richard Kay, of Walmersley, Bury, made reference in his diary to a Samuel and Mary Robinson of Cheetham Hill, who he socialized with. This could suggest a connection between the families. See Richard Kay (1716–1751), Diary, 1737–1751. Chetham's Library. Manchester. A.7.76. Thomas Robinson's son, Thomas the younger, would marry Elizabeth Kay of Bury, giving his son the name Joshua Kay Robinson.
5 Peter Mainwaring's house on King Street was No. 12 when he occupied it, but is No. 35 now. It is the only building still standing from this period of the street's history. It's now a Grade II listed building.
6 Byrom, *The Journal of Elizabeth Byrom*, p. 16.
7 See John Harland, *Collectanea Relating to Manchester and its Neighbourhood, at Various Periods*, vol. II (Manchester: Chetham Society, 1867), pp. 66–76. Harland's account of the concerts in the Chetham Society publication was rediscovered in the twenty-first century by Pauline Nobes, who has worked with a group of musicians to recreate the concerts and stage performances in Manchester. I was made aware of the original concert series through the modern recreations. See *Manchester Baroque*, www.manchesterbaroque.co.uk/about [accessed 8 October 2023].
8 Harland, *Collectanea*, p. 69; original emphasis.
9 Harland, *Collectanea*, p. 71.
10 Brockbank, *Sketches*, p. 23.
11 Brockbank, *Sketches*, p. 23.
12 Jolene Zigarovich, 'Matriarchal Economies: Women Inheriting from Women in Eighteenth-Century Wills, Courts, and Fiction', *Studies in Eighteenth-Century Culture*, 52 (2023), 227–255 (228).
13 Zigarovich, 'Matriarchal Economies', 239.
14 Thomas Apperley married Ann Beswick in September 1756. Hannah's brother also left a bequest to a Beswick living in Ross, his 'kinsman John Beswick of Ross in Herefordshire apothecary'.
15 Some deduction was needed to work out Mary's parentage, so I apologise if I have gone wrong here. As will become clear, Mary had a brother John, who had children called Ann, Henry, Thomas and Frances. An inscription on a grave in Halifax Parish Church, that can only be partially made out, shows a John Greame of Exley dying in 1773, aged sixty-three, and his [illegible, presumably wife] Frances Greame dying in 1775. Above these names on the inscription is another couple, [illegible] who died in 1732, aged forty-seven and his [illegible] Martha Greame who died in 1740. A John Greame married a Martha Earnshaw in Halifax in 1711. Henry Greame, son of Mary's brother John, would name his first-born son John Earnshaw Greame. I've concluded from this that John Greame and Martha Earnshaw were the parents of John

and Mary, and the great-grandparents of John Earnshaw Greame. Some of these Greames will reappear later in the story.

16 John Higson, *The Gorton Historical Recorder, Or, a Concise, Chronological, Ecclesiastical, Municipal, Biographical, and Domestic History of the Chapelry, Illustrating the Rise and Progress of the 'Mesne Manor', and Its Inhabitants, From the Earliest Period to the Present Time* (Droylsden: John Higson, 1852), pp. 82–3.

17 Simon Young, 'John Higson, South Manchester Supernatural', *Beachcombing's Bizarre History Blog,* www.strangehistory.net/puca-ghost-witch-and-fairy-pamphlets/john-higson-south-manchester-supernatural/ [accessed 8 October 2023].

18 Higson, *Gorton Historical Recorder*, p. 7; original emphasis.

19 Joy Margaret Uings, 'Gardens and Gardening in a Fast-Changing Urban Environment: Manchester 1750–1850' (PhD Thesis, Manchester Metropolitan University, 2013), pp. 100–1.

20 Uings, 'Gardens and Gardening', p. 101.

21 *Manchester Mercury*, 27 January 1789.

22 'Writings Missing, Lost or Mislaid', *Manchester Mercury*, 6 December 1791, p. 4. In this rather enigmatic newspaper advertisement, Dr Charles White and Thomas Pickering ask for information relating to the whereabouts of an indenture of mortgage made between John Gorton and Mary Greame of Cheetwood in 1760. The estate in question is Towncroft in Gorton, and it is said to be part of the estate of Hannah Beswick. The advert explains that when Mary Greame married Richard Hopwood, she surrendered her trusteeship of Hannah's estate and all mortgages to Charles White. The problem is that Towncroft wasn't mentioned in Hannah's will (no land in Gorton was), and the indenture was drawn up two years after she died.

23 Hannah's instructions for Sarah Jenkinson were that Charles White and John Whittaker would invest the sum of £200, and then pay the interest received to Sarah for the rest of her life. This legacy differs from those to Esther and Mary, and so I believe the relationship with Sarah was different. It's possible Sarah Jenkinson was Hannah's paid companion, which is why she is offered a continued income after Hannah's death but no personal effects.

OIL OF LAVENDER

1 According to the inventory of Hannah's will, she had issued numerous bonds (debts with interest) in her lifetime. She had loaned money to people we've already met in the story, including Thomas Gorton and Dauntesey Smith, but also to others, including a man called Richard Townsend who owed over £500 (with interest).

2 See Celeste Chamberland, 'Honor, Brotherhood, and the Corporate Ethos of London's Barber-Surgeons' Company, 1570–1640', *Journal of the History of Medicine and Allied Sciences*, 64:3 (July 2009), 300–32.

3 By the early nineteenth century, the figure of the barber-surgeon was treated with distrust and suspicion by many. This distrust was enshrined in the penny dreadful, *The String of Pearls*, in 1846–47, which introduced audiences for the first time to Sweeney Todd, the Demon Barber of Fleet Street.

4 Brockbank, *Sketches*, p. 2.
5 Brockbank, *Sketches*, p. 28.
6 Brockbank, *Sketches*, p. 29.
7 Chaplin, 'Dissection and Display'.
8 Chaplin, 'Dissection and Display'.
9 W. Cheselden, *The Anatomy of the Human Body* (London: N. Cliff & D. Jackson, 1713), p. vii, cited in Chaplin, 'Dissection and Display'. Cheselden's entrepreneurial approach was at odds with the approach taken by the Company of Surgeons, and he was disciplined by the Company in 1715.
10 John Sheldon, *Proposals for a Course of Anatomical, Physiological, and Chirurgical Lectures* (London: printed for the author, *c.* 1778); original in the Countway Library, Harvard (ESTC N12434), cited in Chaplin, 'Dissections and Display'.
11 Richard Kay (1716–1751), Diary, 1737–1751. Chetham's Library, Manchester. A.7.76.
12 See P. Linebaugh, 'The Tyburn Riot Against the Surgeons', in D. Hay, P. Linebaugh, J. G. Rule, E. P. Thompson and C. Winstow (eds), *Albion's Fatal Tree: Crime and Society in Eighteenth Century England* (London: Penguin, 1975), pp. 65–117.
13 A post-mortem differed in theory from a public dissection, as it was intended to determine cause of death or illness, rather than the public display of the corpse as a 'mark of infamy'. More decorous post-mortems might be held in private, but for poorer people with no familial protection, they were often carried out with an audience.
14 Moore, *The Knife Man*, p. 4.
15 John Hunter, *The Case Books of John Hunter FRS*, edited by Elizabeth Allen, J. L. Turk and Sir Reginald Murley (London: Royal Society of Medicine, 1993), pp. 308–9, cited in Moore, *The Knife Man*, p. 37.
16 Chaplin, 'Dissection and Display'.
17 The phrase 'extraordinary collection of specimens' is taken from the Hunterian Museum website: https://hunterianmuseum.org/ [accessed 8 October 2023].
18 Faujas de Saint-Fond, *Travels*, pp. 44–5.
19 Pettigrew, *A History of Egyptian Mummies*, p. 257.
20 Pettigrew, *A History of Egyptian Mummies*, p. 258.
21 *Memoirs of the Manchester Literary and Philosophical Society*, vol. 2 (1789), 366–73. See also Alice Marples, 'Scholarship, Skill and Community: Collections and the Creation of "Provincial" Medical Education in Manchester, 1750–1850', *Journal of the History of Collections*, 33:3 (2021), 505–516.
22 Charles White, *An Account of the Regular Gradation in Man, and in Different Animals and Vegetables; and From the Former to the Latter* (London: C. Dilly, 1799). White's book was dedicated to Sir Richard Clayton, baronet, the author's son-in-law and the grandfather of Richard Clayton Browne-Clayton who claimed to have a coffin in his stable.
23 White, 'Advertisement', in *Regular Gradation*, p. iii.
24 White, *Regular Gradation*, p. 63.
25 Peter M. Dunn, 'Charles White (1728–1813) of Manchester and Fetal Adaptation at Birth', *West of England Medical Journal*, 113:3 (September 2014), Article 2.

26 Marples, 'Scholarship, Skill and Community', 505.
27 Folder: White's Museum, 1932, n.d. Manchester Medical Collection: Biographical Files R-Z. University of Manchester Library. GB 133 MMC/2/WHITEC/4.
28 Folder: White's Museum, 1932, n.d. Manchester Medical Collection: Biographical Files R-Z. University of Manchester Library. GB 133 MMC/2/WHITEC/4. The demise of White's museum is shrouded in mystery. Brockbank claims it was destroyed in a fire, but newspaper reports of the fire at the time specifically state that the museum was saved. When E. Bosdin Leech attempted to find out more in 1932, he simply received a letter back from the hospital (by then St Mary's) stating that none of the specimens were held there anymore.
29 A. Ludlow, 'A Case of Obstructed Deglutition, from a Preternatural Dilatation of and Bag formed in the Pharynx', *Medical Observations and Inquiries by a Society of Physicians in London*, 3 (1764), 85–101, cited in Chaplin, 'Dissection and Display'.
30 Tobias Smollett, *The Letters of Tobias Smollett*, edited by Lewis M. Knapp (Oxford: Clarendon Press, 1970), p. 140, cited in Moore, *The Knife Man*, p. 165.
31 That said, *Body Worlds* has been the subject of a number of investigations surrounding the procurement of bodies for display, including an accusation that they received corpses from prisons, hospitals and psychiatric institutions in Kyrgyzstan without the consent or notification of the deceased's families.

THE PIOUS BAND

1 Friedrich Engels, *The Condition of the Working Class in England*, edited by David McLellan (Oxford and New York: Oxford University Press, 1993), p. 65.
2 Kirby, *Angel Meadow*, p. 13.
3 *Manchester Mercury*, 10 June 1755, p. 1.
4 This example of wages is taken from a 1749 ledger from Arley Hall, Cheshire. See, 'Farm Accounts, 13 January 1749', *Arley Hall Archives, 1750–90*, www.arleyhallarchives.co.uk/farmarley.htm [accessed 8 October 2023].
5 For instance, the average price of a 4lb loaf of bread in London jumped by a full penny in between 1750 and 1751, from 4.7d to 5.52d. See Ronald Sheppard and Edward Newton, *The Story of Bread* (London: Routledge, Kegan and Paul, 1957), p. 168.
6 W. G. Hoskins, 'Harvest Fluctuations and English Economic History, 1620–1759', *Agricultural History Review*, 16 (1968), 15–31 (16).
7 John Bohstedt, *The Politics of Provisions: Food Riots, Moral Economy, and Market Transition in England, c.1550–1850* (London and New York: Routledge, 2010), pp. 103–64.
8 Bohstedt, *The Politics of Provisions*.
9 Michael Nevell, 'From Linen Weaver to Cotton Manufacturer: Manchester During the 17th and 18th Centuries and the Social Archaeology of Industrialisation', *Archaeology North West*, 6:16 (2001–3), 27–44 (31).
10 Nevell, 'From Linen Weaver to Cotton Manufacturer', 33.

11 Nevell, 'From Linen Weaver to Cotton Manufacturer', 34.
12 Romola Jane Davenport, Max Satchell Leigh and Matthew William Shaw-Taylor, 'The Geography of Smallpox in England Before Vaccination: A Conundrum Resolved', *Social Science & Medicine*, 206 (June 2018), 75–85.
13 Bloody flux is a form of dysentery; French pox is syphilis; rising of the lights is a form of lung disease; and St Anthony's Fire is a fungal infection caused by eating infected rye.
14 *Manchester Mercury*, 14 November 1752.
15 *Manchester Mercury*, 27 November 1753.
16 This system of dealing with the poor would continue until the Poor Law Amendment Act 1834, which would decrease the amount of relief offered, worsen conditions in the workhouse and demonize single mothers. *The Times* called the 1834 act 'The Starvation Act', and Charles Dickens memorably drew attention to meagre food rations in *Oliver Twist*.
17 *Manchester Mercury*, 10 June 1755, p. 1.
18 Brockbank, *Sketches*, p. 1.
19 For a detailed exploration of the Infirmary dispute, see J. V. Pickstone and S. V. F. Butler, 'The Politics of Medicine in Manchester, 1788–1792: Hospital Reform and Public Health Services in the Early Industrial City', *Medical History*, 28 (1984), 227–49.

FOUR HUNDRED POUNDS

1 'Funeral of the Countess of Wilton', *Manchester Courier*, 24 December 1858, p. 7.
2 'Interment of Mr Pownall', *Leigh Chronicle and Weekly District Advertiser*, 22 October 1859, p. 3.
3 'Burial of John Robinson Kay', *Bury Times*, 6 April 1872, p. 6.
4 Julian Litten, *The English Way of Death: The Common Funeral since 1450* (London: R. Hale, 1991), pp. 57–84.
5 We have seen this in Britain recently, with the lying in state of Queen Elizabeth II at Westminster Hall, which took place between 14 and 19 September 2022, and the phenomenon of 'The Queue', a ten-mile-long line of people waiting to pay their respects to the dead monarch. Had the body of Queen Elizabeth II not been embalmed and kept in multiple airtight coffins, celebrity queue-jumping would have been the least of the mourners' worries when they entered Westminster Hall.
6 See Litten, *The English Way of Death*, pp. 32–56.
7 *Manchester Courier*, 21 May 1894.
8 See Teerapa Pirohakul, 'The Funeral in England in the Long Eighteenth Century' (PhD Thesis, London School of Economics, 2015), pp. 63–5.
9 Daniel O'Brien, 'The Funeral as an Opportunity for Social Display, 1700–1820, With a Specific Focus on the West Country' (PhD Thesis, University of Bristol, 2018), p. 2.
10 O'Brien, 'The Funeral as an Opportunity for Social Display', p. 66.
11 O'Brien, 'The Funeral as an Opportunity for Social Display', p. 64.
12 O'Brien, 'The Funeral as an Opportunity for Social Display', p. 67.

Notes

13 O'Brien, 'The Funeral as an Opportunity for Social Display', p. 72.
14 *Manchester Mercury*, 15 May 1753. This is not the same establishment as the Swan With Two Necks that survived in Manchester until the end of the twentieth century. This later pub was opened in 1795 on Withy Grove when, presumably, the Market Street establishment mentioned in the 1753 advert had either closed or relocated.
15 *Manchester Mercury*, 26 December 1758.
16 *Manchester Mercury*, 3 August 1762.
17 Pirohakul, 'The Funeral in England', p. 58.
18 Thomas Doolittle (1632?–1707), *A Sermon on Eyeing of Eternity, So That It May Have Its Due Influence upon Us in All We Do*, 2nd edn (London, 1755), p. 74, cited in Jolene Zigarovich, 'Preserved Remains: Embalming Practices in Eighteenth-Century England', *Eighteenth-Century Life*, 33:3 (Fall 2009), 65–104 (72).
19 Francis Bancroft, *A True Copy of the Remarkable Last Will and Testament of Mr Francis Bancroft, Citizen and Draper of London* (London: J. Peele, 1728), p. 6, cited in Zigarovich, 'Preserved Remains', 75.
20 See Zigarovich, 'Preserved Remains', 77.
21 All these examples are found in Zigarovich, 'Preserved Remains', 77.
22 Thomas Greenhill, *NEKPOKHΔEIA; Or, the Art of Embalming; Wherein Is Shewn the Right of Burial, and Funeral Ceremonies, Especially That of Preserving Bodies After the Egyptian Method. Together With an Account of the Egyptian Mummies, Pyramids, Subterranean Vaults and Lamps, and Their Opinion of the Metempsychosis, the Cause of Their Embalming. As Also a Geographical Description of Egypt, the Rise and Course of the Nile, the Temper, Constitution and Physic of the Inhabitants, Their Inventions, Arts, Sciences, Stupendous Works and Sepulchres, and Other Curious Observations Any Ways Relating to the Physiology and Knowledge of This Art* (London: Thomas Greenhill, 1705), pp. 178–9; original emphasis. It should be noted that Greenhill was a surgeon, and his book was crowdfunded through 'subscriptions' that were, as the front material reveals, almost entirely bought by surgeons and apothecaries.
23 R. Campbell, *The London Tradesman: Being a Compendious View of all the Trades, Professions, Arts, both Liberal and Mechanic, now practised in the Cities of London and Westminster* (London, 1747), pp. 329–30, cited in Paul S. Fritz, 'The Undertaking Trade in England: Its Origins and Early Development, 1660–1830', *Eighteenth-Century Studies*, 28:2 (Winter 1994–5), 241–53.
24 *Funeral Discipline; Or, the Character of Strip-corps the Dead-monger: Written According to the Instructions of Paul Meagre, Once Mourner in Chief to the Funeral Undertaker* (1701), cited by Daniel O'Brien in 'Undertakers and the Body in Eighteenth Century Satire', an online talk for *Romancing the Gothic*, 31 October 2022.
25 Matthew D. Turner, '"Forbidden Fish": Did King Henry I Die of Lamprey Poisoning?', *Cureus*, 15:5 (May 2023), www.ncbi.nlm.nih.gov/pmc/articles/PMC10281476/ [accessed 8 October 2023].
26 Zigarovich, 'Preserved Remains', 67.

27 'What is Embalming?', *Coop*, www.coop.co.uk/funeralcare/advice/what-is-embalming [accessed 8 October 2023].
28 'Life and Death in Manchester: Excavations Along the Second City Crossing', https://diggreatermanchester.files.wordpress.com/2021/12/gmpr29–life-and-death-in-manchester.pdf [accessed 8 October 2023].

UNREMARKABLE

1 Samuel Bamford, *Bamford's Passages in the Life of a Radical and Early Days in Two Volumes*, vol. 1, edited by Henry Dunckley (London: T. Fisher Unwin, 1893), p. 90.
2 Bamford, *Passages in the Life of a Radical*, p. 91. Samuel Bamford was a friend and colleague of James Dronsfield. I have to wonder, when Dronsfield published his account of the Legend of Birchen Bower, did his friend realize that Madame Beswick was related to his old childhood pal Sam?
3 Clare Hartwell, *Manchester*, Pevsner Architectural Guides (London: Penguin Books, 2001), p. 71.
4 The zoo at Belle Vue gardens continued as a popular attraction into the twentieth century, becoming well known for its elephants. The most famous of the Belle Vue elephants was Maharajah, who arrived in 1872. After Maharajah destroyed the railway carriage that was supposed to be transporting him, he had to walk (with his keeper, Lorenzo Lawrence) from Edinburgh to Belle Vue, which garnered a lot of media attention. Maharajah died in 1882, and his skeleton was displayed in the Belle Vue Natural History Museum. It is now part of the collection at the Manchester Museum.
5 See Thomas Swindells, *Manchester Streets and Manchester Men* (Manchester: J. E. Cornish, 1908), pp. 149–53.
6 Cucumbers, in particular, were deeply unpopular during Hannah's lifetime. Samuel Johnson, writing in 1773, referred to them as 'good for nothing'.
7 One line of descent that has been claimed for this family is from Ivo de Taillebois, Earl of Anjou, who came over to England with William I in 1066. This version of the family tree (which is admittedly contested) has Ivo's great-grandson, Nicholas Fitz-Gilbert de Tailbois, being granted lands at Radcliffe, Lancashire, in the twelfth century and styling himself 'Nicholas de Radcliffe'.

EPILOGUE

1 Topic: Tesco built on my grandfathers grave in Cheetham Hill, *Manchester Forum*, 12 March 2013, www.manchester-forum.co.uk/index.php?topic=8100.0 [accessed 11 October 2023].
2 'Notables, Page 1', *Manchester General Cemetery Transcription Project*, www.mgctp.co.uk/notables-page-1 [accessed 11 October 2023].
3 An amendment was made to the Act shortly before it was passed in parliament, stating that authorities should 'have regard to the desirability of' disposing of a body according to a person's wishes or religious beliefs, even if the decision was taken that those wishes had to be disregarded.

Select bibliography

Alberti, Samuel J. M. M., 'Placing Nature: Natural History Collections and Their Owners in Nineteenth-Century Provincial England', *The British Journal for the History of Science*, 35:3 (September 2002), 291–311.

—, *Nature and Culture Objects, Disciplines and the Manchester Museum* (Manchester: Manchester University Press, 2012).

Ashton, Thomas, *Visits to the Museum of the Manchester Natural History Society* (Manchester: Manchester Natural History Society, 1857).

Bamford, Samuel, *Bamford's Passages in the Life of a Radical and Early Days in Two Volumes*, vol. 1, edited by Henry Dunckley (London: T. Fisher Unwin, 1893).

Bohstedt, John, *The Politics of Provisions: Food Riots, Moral Economy, and Market Transition in England, c.1550–1850* (London and New York: Routledge, 2010).

Bondeson, Jan, *Buried Alive: The Terrifying History of Our Most Primal Fear* (London and New York: W. W. Norton and Co., 2001).

Brockbank, E. M., *Sketches of the Lives and Work of the Honorary Medical Staff of the Manchester Infirmary, from its Foundation in 1752 to 1830 when it became the Royal Infirmary* (Manchester: Manchester University Press, 1904).

Brunvand, Jan Harold, *The Vanishing Hitchhiker: American Urban Legends and Their Meanings* (New York: W. W. Norton and Co., 1981).

Butterworth, Edwin, *Historical Sketches of Oldham* (Oldham: J. Hirst, 1856).

Byrom, Elizabeth, *The Journal of Elizabeth Byrom in 1745*, edited by Richard Parkinson (Manchester: Chetham Society, 1857).

Campbell, Thomas, *Reprint of Mr Campbell's Letter to Mr Brougham, on the Subject of a London University, which Appeared in The Times of Feb. 9: Together with Suggestions which Appeared in the April Number of the New Monthly Magazine* (London: Longman, Hurst, Rees, Orme, Brown, and Green, 1825).

Chadwick, William, *Reminiscences of a Chief Constable* (Manchester: John Heywood, 1900).

Chamberland, Celeste, 'Honor, Brotherhood, and the Corporate Ethos of London's Barber-Surgeons' Company, 1570–1640', *Journal of the History of Medicine and Allied Sciences*, 64:3 (July 2009), 300–32.

Chaplin, Simon, 'Dissection and Display in Eighteenth-Century London', in Piers Mitchell (ed.), *Anatomical Dissection in Enlightenment England and Beyond Autopsy, Pathology and Display* (London: Routledge, 2012), pp. 95–114.

Select bibliography

Charlton, Henry Buckley, *Portrait of a University, 1851–1951: To Commemorate the Centenary of Manchester University* (Manchester: Manchester University Press, 1951).

Crawford, Joseph, '"A Tale of Plague": Anti-Medical Sentiment and Epidemic Disease in Early Victorian Popular Gothic Fiction', in Nicole C. Dittmer and Sophie Raine (eds), *Penny Dreadfuls and the Gothic: Investigations of Pernicious Tales of Terror* (Cardiff: University of Wales Press, 2023), pp. 114–36.

Darwin, Charles, *The Variation of Animals and Plants Under Domestication*, vol. II (London: John Murray, 1868).

Davenport, Romola Jane, Max Satchell, Leigh Matthew and William Shaw-Taylor, 'The Geography of Smallpox in England Before Vaccination: A Conundrum Resolved', *Social Science & Medicine*, 206 (June 2018), 75–85.

Defoe, Daniel, *A Tour Thro' the Whole Island of Great Britain, Divided into Circuits or Journies* (London: JM Dent and Co, 1927).

Dobson, Jessie, 'Some Eighteenth Century Experiments in Embalming', *Journal of the History of Medicine and Allied Sciences*, 8:4 (October 1953), 431–41.

Dronsfield, James, *Ouselwood, or A Gathering of Old Chums* (Oldham: John Albinson, Ltd., 1921).

Dunn, Peter M., 'Charles White (1728–1813) of Manchester and Fetal Adaptation at Birth', *West of England Medical Journal*, 113:3 (September 2014), Article 2.

Engels, Friedrich, *The Condition of the Working Class in England*, edited by David McLellan (Oxford and New York: Oxford University Press, 1993).

Exell, Karen, 'Covering the Mummies at the Manchester Museum: A Discussion of Individual Agendas Within the Human Remains Debate', in Howard Williams and Melanie Giles (eds), *Archaeologists and the Dead: Mortuary Archaeology and Contemporary Society* (Oxford: Oxford University Press, 2016), pp. 233–49.

—, 'Domination and Desire: The Paradox of Egyptian Mummies in Museums', in Penelope Harvey (ed.), *Objects and Materials: A Routledge Companion* (London: Routledge, 2013), pp. 144–55.

Faujas de Saint-Fond, Barthélemy, *Travels in England, Scotland, and the Hebrides; Undertaken for the Purpose of Examining the State of the Arts, the Sciences, Natural History and Manners in Great Britain* (London: James Ridgeway, 1799).

Frith, Henry, *Haunted Ancestral Homes*, edited by J. Murphy (Morrisville: Lulu.com, 2017).

Fritz, Paul S., 'The Undertaking Trade in England: Its Origins and Early Development, 1660–1830', *Eighteenth-Century Studies*, 28:2 (Winter 1994–95), 241–53.

Goldsmith, Oliver, *The History of The Earth and Animated Nature, With Copious Notes and an Appendix by Captain Thomas Brown*, edited by Thomas Brown (Glasgow: A. Fullarton and Co., 1832).

Greenhill, Thomas, *NEKPOKHΔEIA; Or, the Art of Embalming; Wherein Is Shewn the Right of Burial, and Funeral Ceremonies, Especially That of Preserving Bodies After the Egyptian Method. Together With an Account of the Egyptian Mummies, Pyramids, Subterranean Vaults and Lamps, and Their Opinion of the Metempsychosis, the Cause of Their Embalming. As Also a Geographical Description of Egypt, the Rise and Course of the Nile, the Temper, Constitution and Physic of the Inhabitants, Their Inventions, Arts, Sciences, Stupendous*

Works and Sepulchres, and Other Curious Observations Any Ways Relating to the Physiology and Knowledge of This Art (London: Thomas Greenhill, 1705).

Harland, John, *Collectanea Relating to Manchester and its Neighbourhood, at Various Periods*, vol. II (Manchester: Chetham Society, 1867).

Hartwell, Clare, *Manchester*, Pevsner Architectural Guides (London: Penguin Books, 2001).

Head, George, *A Home Tour Through the Manufacturing Districts of England, in the Summer of 1835* (London: John Murray, 1836).

Henry, William, 'A Tribute to the Memory of the Late President of the Literary and Philosophical Society of Manchester', *Memoirs of the Literary and Philosophical Society of Manchester*, second series, vol. III (1819), 204–40.

Higson, John, *The Gorton Historical Recorder, Or, a Concise, Chronological, Ecclesiastical, Municipal, Biographical, and Domestic History of the Chapelry, Illustrating the Rise and Progress of the 'Mesne Manor', and Its Inhabitants, From the Earliest Period to the Present Time* (Droylsden: John Higson, 1852).

Holmes, Rachel, *The Hottentot Venus: The Life and Death of Sarah Baartman* (London: Bloomsbury, 2007).

Hoskins, W. G., 'Harvest Fluctuations and English Economic History, 1620–1759', *Agricultural History Review*, 16 (1968), 15–31.

Ingram, John H., *The Haunted Homes and Family Traditions of Great Britain* (London: Gibbings & Co., 1897).

Kay, Richard, *The Diary of Richard Kay, 1716–51 of Baldingstone, Near Bury: A Lancashire Doctor*, edited by W. Brockbank and F. Kenworth (Manchester: Chetham Society, 1968).

Kirby, Dean, *Angel Meadow: Victorian Britain's Most Savage Slum* (Barnsley: Pen and Sword Books, 2016).

Kitson, Peter, 'The Strange Case of Dr White and Mr De Quincey: Manchester, Medicine and Romantic Theories of Biological Racism', *Romanticism*, 17:3 (October 2011), 278–87.

Kohl, Johann Georg, *England, Wales and Scotland* (London: Chapman and Hall, 1844).

Lees, Colin and Alex Roberton, 'Early Students and the "University of the Busy": the Quay Street Years of Owens College, 1851–1870', *Bulletin of the John Rylands Library* (1997), 161–94.

Linebaugh, P., 'The Tyburn Riot Against the Surgeons' in D. Hay, P. Linebaugh, J. G. Rule, E. P. Thompson and C. Winstow (eds), *Albion's Fatal Tree: Crime and Society in Eighteenth Century England* (London: Penguin, 1975), pp. 65–117.

Litten, Julian, *The English Way of Death: The Common Funeral since 1450* (London: R. Hale, 1991).

Love, Benjamin, *Manchester As It Is* (Manchester: Love and Barton, 1839).

Ludlam, Harry, *The Mummy of Birchen Bower and Other True Ghost Stories* (Slough: W. Foulsham and Co., 1985 [1966]).

Marples, Alice, 'Scholarship, Skill and Community: Collections and the Creation of 'Provincial' Medical Education in Manchester, 1750–1850', *Journal of the History of Collections*, 33:3 (2021), 505–16.

Maw, Peter, 'Provincial Merchants in Eighteenth-Century England: The "Great Oaks" of Manchester', *The English Historical Review*, 136:580 (June 2021), 568–618.

Moore, Wendy, *The Knife Man: Blood, Body Snatching, and the Birth of Modern Surgery* (New York: Broadway Books, 2005).
Musson, A. E. and E. Robinson, 'Science and Industry in the Late Eighteenth Century', *The Economic History Review*, new series, 13:2 (1960), 222–44.
Nevell, Michael, 'From Linen Weaver to Cotton Manufacturer: Manchester During the 17th and 18th Centuries and the Social Archaeology of Industrialisation', *Archaeology North West*, 6:16 (2001–3), 27–44.
Nicholson, Francis, 'The Old Manchester Natural History Society and its Museum', in *Memoirs and Proceedings of the Manchester Literary and Philosophical Society (Manchester Memoirs)*, vol. 58 (1913–14) (Manchester: Manchester Literary and Philosophical Society, 1915), pp. 1–15.
O'Brien, Daniel, 'The Funeral as an Opportunity for Social Display, 1700–1820, With a Specific Focus on the West Country' (PhD Thesis, University of Bristol, 2018).
Osborn, Matthew, '"The Weirdest of All Undertakings": The Land and the Early Industrial Revolution in Oldham, England', *Environmental History*, 8:2 (April 2003), 246–69.
Pettigrew, Thomas, *A History of Egyptian Mummies, and an Account of the Worship and Embalming of the Sacred Animals by the Egyptians; with Remarks on the Funeral Ceremonies of Different Nations, and Observations on the Mummies of the Canary Islands, of the Ancient Peruvians, Burman Priests, etc.* (London: Longman, Rees, Orme, Brown, Green and Longman, 1834).
Pevsner, Nikolaus, *Lancashire I: The Industrial and Commercial South* (London: Penguin Books, 1969).
Pickstone, J. V. and S. V. F. Butler, 'The Politics of Medicine in Manchester, 1788–1792: Hospital Reform and Public Health Services in the Early Industrial City', *Medical History*, 28 (1984), 227–49.
Pirohakul, Teerapa, 'The Funeral in England in the Long Eighteenth Century' (PhD Thesis, London School of Economics, 2015).
Price, Campbell, *Golden Mummies of Egypt: Interpreting Identities from the Graeco-Roman Period* (Manchester: Manchester University Press, 2023).
Quincey, Thomas de, *Selected Writings of Thomas de Quincey*, edited by Philip van Doren Stern (New York: The Modern Library).
Riggs, Christina, *Unwrapping Ancient Egypt* (London: Bloomsbury, 2014).
Roscoe, H. E., *Record of Work Done in the Chemical Department of the Owens College 1857–1887* (London: Macmillan, 1887).
Sheppard, Ronald and Edward Newton, *The Story of Bread* (London: Routledge, Kegan and Paul, 1957).
Sitwell, Edith, *English Eccentrics* (London: Faber & Faber, 1958 [1933]).
Stienne, Angela, *Mummified: The Stories Behind Egyptian Mummies in Museums* (Manchester: Manchester University Press, 2022).
Sugg, Richard, *Mummies, Cannibals and Vampires: The History of Corpse Medicine from the Renaissance to the Victorians* (London and New York: Routledge, 2011).
Swindells, Thomas, *Manchester Streets and Manchester Men* (Manchester: J. E. Cornish, 1908).
Thackray, Arnold, 'Natural Knowledge in Cultural Context: The Manchester Mode', *The American Historical Review*, 79:3 (June 1974), 672–709.

Uings, Joy Margaret, 'Gardens and Gardening in a Fast-Changing Urban Environment: Manchester 1750–1850' (PhD Thesis, Manchester Metropolitan University, 2013).

Wasson, Sara, 'Gothic Cities and Suburbs, 1880–Present', in Glennis Byron and Dale Townshend (eds), *The Gothic World* (London and New York: Routledge, 2014), pp. 132–42.

Webb, Katherine, '"The Most Stupid Place Under the Sun": Medical Practice and Professional Aspirations in the Industrial Town, 1820–60', *Bulletin of the John Rylands Library*, 87:1 (March 2005), 57–87.

White, Charles, *An Account of the Regular Gradation in Man, and in Different Animals and Vegetables; and From the Former to the Latter* (London: C. Dilly, 1799).

Williamson, William Crawford, *Reminiscences of a Yorkshire Naturalist* (London: George Redway, 1896).

Zigarovich, Jolene, 'Preserved Remains: Embalming Practices in Eighteenth-Century England', *Eighteenth-Century Life*, 33:3 (Fall 2009), 65–104.

—, 'Matriarchal Economies: Women Inheriting from Women in Eighteenth-Century Wills, Courts, and Fiction', *Studies in Eighteenth-Century Culture*, 52 (2023), 227–255.

Index

Index

Index

Index

Index